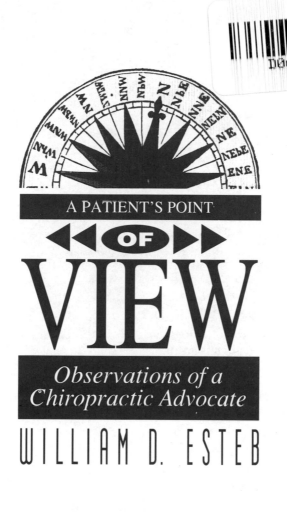

A PATIENT'S POINT

◄◄ **OF** ►►

VIEW

*Observations of a
Chiropractic Advocate*

WILLIAM D. ESTEB

Published by Orion Associates

Published by
Orion Associates
P.O. Box 38218
Colorado Springs, CO 80937

Cover design by Buffalo Brothers, Inc.
Manufactured in the United States of America

Esteb, William D., 1952–

A Patient's Point of View
Observations of a Chiropractic Advocate / William D. Esteb
ISBN 0-9631711-0-0

For my son Eric Ross Esteb, who is a constant reminder that miracles are all around us.

CONTENTS

FOREWORD

Thomas Savage wrote in his Montana novel, *The Corner of Rife and Pacific*, "My father's a chiropractor. He meant to be a doctor, but never made it."

It is Savage's perception, shared by so many others, that is at the root of the barrier to the acceptance and utilization of chiropractic today. It is not competition from the chiropractor down the block or the medical physician. Our enemy is the opinions, or lack of opinions, of a large percentage of people who do not understand; who have not been educated to the dimensions of chiropractic.

This, along with the fact that we so easily get wrapped up in technique, philosophy, or management dogma, causes us to forget what patients really want.

Bill Esteb, a non-chiropractor, fully armed in chiropractic through a genesis with Renaissance International, the adjusting table, and seminar audiences, asks us to "get real." He observes that chiropractors live in a subculture. Our philosophy and distorted world-view endangers our ability to survive and thrive; to realize our chiropractic goals for a better world.

Mr. Esteb travels through many "moments of truth" so we can enjoy healthier patient relationships and empower our patients. He explores the role of patient feedback in the achievement of our individual practice dreams.

Read and be prepared to leave your comfort zone and adventure into new territories as you better appreciate what makes today's new patient tick.

James R. Milliron, D.C.

INTRODUCTION

If you've been at chiropractic for a while and venture into Bill Esteb's book, be prepared to spend. Time, money, and energy will beg for your attention when you compare your present place with the vision Bill is suggesting here. If you've been in the practice of the science, philosophy, and art of chiropractic for any time at all, you will find little difficulty in appreciating and implementing the things which chiropractic advocate Esteb recommends.

If, on the other hand, you are new in practice or new to the vision of a safer, sounder world arrived at through the deductive thought and understanding of chiropractic, you might wonder, "What more does this guy want from me?" It is for you, who finds this book overwhelming, that this introduction is written.

There is no doubt that should you find this book discouraging in any way it is because you do not have the vision or it has grown fuzzy. Maybe you're the scientist who says, "Results speak for themselves." And they might, but results alone do not carry others over the threshold into your office or the offices of other chiropractors.

Results are what patients and insurance companies pay for, and expect. What does it take to urge patients to refer others? Knowledge, excitement, understanding, being cared for, love, appreciation, and approval are but a few. Get the idea? You cannot leave one stone unturned in your quest to establish a place of healing where all will continue to feel welcome and equipped to tell others.

Where are you? Established, entrenched, and excited? Grown stale and contemplating getting out? In pursuit of the D.C. degree or anticipating your grand opening? No matter! You'll find plenty of fuel for the fire within this book by chiropractic advocate and friend Bill Esteb. Get going!

Will Tickel, D.C.

PROLOGUE

When I was a child I remember asking my parents at the dinner table how my stomach knew which compartment to put the food in as I ate it. "How does it know to put the corn in the corn compartment and the hamburger in the hamburger compartment?" I asked, eager to learn.

I've been asking questions about how my body functions ever since.

The questions since 1981 have primarily involved chiropractic. That's when Dr. Joseph Flesia and Dr. Guy Riekeman of Renaissance International asked me to write their patient education videos. Helping to create the classic Peter Graves, Russell Erhardt, D.C., and Jayne Kennedy videos while I was working at International Media Systems was an exciting, collaborative experience.

In 1987, Dr. Flesia invited me to begin contributing to a monthly Renaissance publication titled *New Dimensions*. About a dozen of my articles were published over the years, and I still continue the discipline of writing a 1300-word article once a month. The articles have been a way of thinking out loud and arranging the "compartments" of my mind as I continue to grow in my chiropractic understanding.

This volume is a compilation of some of my favorites. As you will see, patient education, communications, and the value of a chiropractic lifestyle are consistent themes.

I hope this collection can be a source of inspiration and motivation for you as you persevere in the detection, elimination, and prevention of the Vertebral Subluxation Complex.

GET REAL

You live in a subculture called chiropractic. It separates you from the patients you serve. It insulates you from fully understanding and reading their motives. It distorts your perceptions of the world. It endangers your ability to survive and thrive in the tumultuous years ahead. You are like the fish who is in water, but doesn't know he's wet.

Noticing people's posture when you're shopping at the mall is not normal behavior!

Philosophy, technique, and procedures are important. Yet, until you know what your patients are thinking and saying about your practice, every new patient approach is a guess or a gimmick. In the process of speculating why patients do what they do, you sabotage your self-worth, risk your professional reputation, and project a lack of confidence that new patients, who are extremely sensitive and apprehensive, can read loud and clear. You are inadvertently saying and doing things, or *not* saying and doing things, that are causing negative word-of-mouth advertising about you and your practice. These patient "pet peeves" are rarely centered around issues like your adjusting style, amount of time spent with patients, your staff, or type of adjusting table you use. More often the issues are more subtle, and quickly correctable—if you knew what they were.

The temptation is to remain isolated and protect our fragile egos from the truth. We kid ourselves and think that by somehow ignoring the truth or "keeping a professional distance" from patients that we can avoid the personal blame of few new patients or poor compliance. It's not just in

17

chiropractic. Restaurant chefs avoid taking the 12 steps over to the dishwasher to see what culinary masterpieces of their's aren't being eaten. Seminar speakers avoid taking phone calls from attendees. Airline pilots avoid contact with passengers after a particularly poor landing.

Get real.

Look to the cause

When the boss is in denial, the business loses its rudder and challenges strike the practice, seemingly without cause or obvious solution. Unexplained high staff turnover occurs. A lingering illness diminishes productivity. A few unappreciative patients ruin an otherwise wonderful day. The doctor becomes increasingly isolated and uncommunicative. The practice becomes a tiresome treadmill without fulfillment or purpose. Caught in this vortex of uncertainty and frustration, the doctor (like patients) is tempted to become focused outside, at the symptom, instead of the cause.

"Maybe I should hire an associate?"

"I'm thinking about building my own building."

"What do you think about this new advertising program I'm considering?"

"I think I need another vacation."

"I'm going to switch management consultants."

"I'm looking at moving my office."

As a non-D.C., I'm always amazed by doctors who step on the dollar bills to pick up the nickels. Doctors who are so close to chiropractic they can't see its incredible simplicity, attractiveness, and compelling power. Doctors who get in the way of chiropractic. Doctors who inadvertently cover the brilliance, subdue the excitement, and make chiropractic pedestrian and unattractive.

Because we are afraid.

We are afraid to ask. We are afraid to confront. We are afraid of change. We are afraid to try. We are afraid our spouse will leave us. We are afraid our children will hate us. We are afraid of what our friends and neighbors will think. We are afraid of the bank. We are afraid of insurance companies. We are afraid to take post X-rays. We are afraid to call the patient after the first adjustment. We are afraid to know what our patients really think. We are afraid to take a stand. We are afraid to make a 100% commitment. We are afraid to be wrong. We are afraid to reveal our chiropractic identity. We are afraid we won't be able to pay our bills. We are afraid of our own potential. We are afraid someone will find out who we really are. We are afraid of accountability.

What many chiropractic patients meet on their first visit is a frightened doctor. Like themselves. You can't necessarily tell it in the doctor's handshake. The voice seems well-modulated and controlled. However, there's something subtle about the doctor that seems timid, weak, reserved, and lacking self confidence. It sets the tone for the doctor/patient relationship and even interferes with the healing process.

What patients want

Besides the pain relief for which patients seek your office, patients want passion. Not necessarily that of a charismatic cult leader. They want conviction. They want to see commitment. In a world of constant change they want to see confidence and self-reliance. They want to see energy. Not the raw, hyper kind, but the efficient, purposeful kind. They want to see pride. They want a mentor. They want to see a living testimonial of the power and "rightness" of chiropractic.

In an era of antibiotics, organ transplants, and DNA splicing, chiropractic may be too "low-tech" to be fashionable. No one said it would be easy to explain the fact that patients heal themselves (as long as there isn't any interference). In a culture that is drawn to accept technological innovations that make health appear to be something that comes from the outside (drugs and surgery), it requires sensitivity and creativity to communicate effectively. Something difficult to do if you doubt chiropractic, question whether structural changes are possible, don't see any value of chiropractic care beyond merely symptomatic relief, or will only recommend what an insurance company will pay for without putting up a fight.

Efferent and afferent

For too long this profession has focused on the content and presentation of the message sent to (or at) patients. Finding the perfect report of findings, telephone scripts, "Rambo" recall programs, admitting forms, and collection strategies has become the focus of many offices. While all these communication efforts may be necessary, many doctors forget that effective communication is a loop: a message is sent and a feedback loop confirms the message was decoded properly. Most offices ignore this feedback loop except for the crudest statistical measures such as patient volume, patient visit average, and collections. This would be like McDonald's attempting to measure customer satisfaction by weighing the contents of their garbage cans!

Whether you like to admit it or not, your patients control compliance, referrals, and word-of-mouth advertising about your practice. Since patients do what they do, because they think what they think, it's important to know what they're thinking. It can help you predict their behavior—which is helpful since they write your paycheck each month!

Want to have more fun? Confront the great unknown. Find out what psychological and attitudinal adjustments your patients need as you render their spinal adjustments. If you don't know what needs to be modified in their cranium, you'll have few opportunities modify the space between their occiput and coccyx. Get a new sensitivity to the language called Patientese.

1. Hold regular patient focus groups. Invite a group of six or seven patients that share something in common (health attitude, symptomatology, how they pay for care, age, etc.) to lunch. Pick their brains about aspects of your office such as procedures, staffing, environment, bedside manner, and other factors that influence their perceptions, compliance, and ultimately their ability to refer others.

2. Call patients after their first adjustment. Prepare a response in advance to anything they might say. Be ready to explain why they may be sore. Help them integrate this new thing called chiropractic into their lives.

3. Ask patients on their first visit what they hope to do with their newfound health. Find out what's important to them. Discover their key values. Find out what will most likely motivate them to follow through with your recommendations. It's not to normalize their spinal biomechanics or improve their posture!

4. During your clinical routine ask patients, "I was wondering, how do you describe what goes on in our office to others?" Then listen to their answer as if your practice depended upon it. Because it does! As they practice their referral dialogue in front of you, note areas where their chiropractic education is still lacking. Then, get to work on subsequent visits.

5. Ask patients what they think the general public's greatest fear or apprehension is about consulting a chiropractic office. Chances are they may still harbor this concern, pass it along to others, or are ineffective in explaining or defending this notion to others they meet. Find out. "So, when you talk to others about chiropractic, how do you explain this fear or apprehension isn't true?"

Not knowing the truth holds us in bondage. Things happen to us and we become bystanders to our own lives. While it may be painful, the truth sets us free. Without the truth, patients suffer and chiropractic will suffer. Take a deep breath and discover how the world clears a path for the fearless. ■

CLEARING A PATIENT'S INTERNAL DIALOGUE

Your patient seems distant. He asks a question at the conclusion of your report of findings that you answered during the first three minutes. He doesn't follow through. He says one thing and does something completely different, even counterproductive to your recommendations.

Everyone hears voices

Unexplainable behavior is often the result of something the communication industry refers to as internal dialogue. It's that little voice we each hear as we go about our lives. This "self-talk" keeps us in touch with our belief system as we constantly monitor the world around us. It helps us form opinions and gives us ways to organize our thoughts so we can respond with appropriate actions. Of particular interest is the internal dialogue of the new patient.

Responding to the internal dialogue of new patients is the largest non-clinical challenge facing today's doctor of chiropractic. It's absent when we're relaxed, talking with old friends when our defenses are down, yet it dominates the landscape of a new doctor/patient relationship—especially in chiropractic. Listen in on the internal dialogue of a typical new patient:

"What will the office look like? Do I trust the doctor? Will it hurt? Will I have to take off my clothes? Will I have to go for the rest of my life? How long will it take? Will there be other patients like me in the office? How much will it cost? I hope my insurance covers this. I hope he doesn't break my neck. Aunt Martha said chiropractic helped her. I better not tell my doctor I went to a chiropractor. Will it be expensive? Will I have to wait a long time? What if it doesn't work? If Bob ever finds out I fell for one of those charismatic chiropractors..."

This chatter will go on and on inside the mind of the new patient unless there is an organized method to intervene in this distracting and sometimes self-limiting internal dialogue.

As a chiropractic doctor, among your most frequent battles are those needed to identify and neutralize the internal dialogue among your patients. Dealing with this issue successfully is a common denominator of growing, enthusiastic, and effective practices. And while there are often common areas, every patient walks into your life with a different set of matching luggage containing a lifetime of attitudes, perceptions, and opinions about their health, you, and chiropractic in general.

It happened to me

As a new chiropractic patient, I walked into an empty waiting room at 10:00 a.m. on a Thursday morning in early 1981. Today I understand that Thursdays are often not fully utilized in many chiropractic offices. But as a newcomer walking into a doctor's empty office in the middle of prime business hours was extremely unsettling. Ever enter a restaurant during the dinner hour and find it empty? I almost ended my first chiropractic experience before it began. The way in which the staff member set up my appointment contributed to some very unnecessary internal dialogue; it had not been communicated that "Thursdays are reserved for new patients so we can devote 100% of our attention..." Without the sensitivity needed to recognize my concerns and perceptions as a new patient, the doctor had to work harder to assure me that he was successful, had other patients, and that I had chosen the right doctor. By ignoring my internal dialogue and not being sensitive to my first impressions, the office had to overcome my doubts about the wisdom of even beginning chiropractic care! Needless to say, it is not an ideal position in which to begin a relationship with a new patient.

The solution

I know of only one way to remove negative internal dialogue and begin the process of reversing the misconceptions and objections to chiropractic care: a committed effort to over-communicate with patients. When combined with an aggressive patient education program, the problems of negative internal dialogue can be prevented before they begin.

Over-communication starts with your yellow page advertising, continues through the first telephone contact with a new patient, and never ends. It requires a conscious effort to anticipate and freely volunteer information, rather than waiting for patients to garner the courage or insight to ask their questions. Chiropractic suffers from so much misunderstanding and lack of acceptance, a primary strategy to reverse the process must include over-communication and being ultra-sensitive to the internal dialogue patients might be experiencing as they begin and continue to receive care in your office.

I'd heard chiropractic is expensive

While an adjustment that unlocks one's human potential may be worth a million dollars, that's not what the market will bear. Fees are a factor in any chiropractic decision because the word on the street is that chiropractic is expensive. Decide on a strategy to overcome this misconception–or affirm it. Offices reluctant or unable to articulate their fee structure and its fairness over the telephone are often the same offices with the largest collection problems. Patients who ask about the cost are not necessarily shopping for the lowest rates. They're simply responding to their internal dialogue.

The same holds true for X-rays. The word on the street has it that after falling for a charismatic doctor, you'll be charged for a lot of expensive X-rays. Or so many will be taken, you'll glow. Concerns about radiation exposure can be guises to cover up fear about the quantity and cost of the X-rays. Are your X-ray charges fair? Do you volunteer an explanation of how you minimize X-ray exposure?

Variations on these internal dialogue issues surface during my focus groups with chiropractic patients. It is often the lack of a communication plan by the doctor and staff that creates the most potentially damaging internal dialogue. Every office should identify sources of potential patient internal dialogue by keeping a record of questions asked by new patients and then developing a strategy for anticipating and volunteering answers to those questions before they are asked.

If you're getting a lot of questions from patients, you probably have compliance problems too. In those practices where successful patient education is a primary objective and anticipating patient questions before they are asked is a full-time job of the staff, compliance, retention, and long-term rehabilitative care are also found.

Service to others is the highest calling to which any of us can aspire. And the highest form of service is anticipating someone else's needs. It raises their self-esteem. It clears the air. And it is the basis of trusting, long-term relationships. ■

OUT OF
THE CLOSET

I have the occasion to travel frequently, and when I meet people on airplanes the inevitable question of what I do often arises. It's a common question asked with sincere interest. I confess that my response has not always been complete.

During my early exposure to chiropractic, while I was researching and writing the Renaissance patient education videotapes, I would enthusiastically reveal my newfound understanding and appreciation for chiropractic. Excited by the simple logic of chiropractic principles and inspired by the improvement of my own health, I was quick to gush my endorsement for chiropractic.

It didn't take long before the polite "uh-huhs" and mild curiosity of my close circle of friends was replaced with hostile questions and raised eyebrows. My reputation and judgment were somehow in question by my association with "quarpractors." It was as if I had fallen prey to some charismatic, money-hungry cult! After submitting to enough abuse, I found myself couching my response with explanations like, "I work with doctors," or "I'm involved in patient education." Only if there were follow up questions did I reveal my chiropractic identity.

Now I'm ashamed of my avoidance. I'm sharing my experience as a cleansing confession and to help keep others, many others in chiropractic I'm discovering, from doing the same thing. No more side-stepping!

C.A. stands for Chiropractic Assistant, not "Closet Advocate." And D.C. stands for Doctor of Chiropractic, not "Defensive Crusader." Those who have created new paths and changed the direction of humanity have always been persecuted: Christ, Gandhi, Martin Luther King, etc. And regardless of the reception these leaders received, the truth has prevailed. By avoiding being identified with chiropractic, I was inadvertently admitting that chiropractic's detractors were right. Those who posses the truth have the obligation to do everything possible to share it. No one lights a lamp and covers it with a bowl!

Making a difference

I made this observation while reading *Dedication and Leadership* by Douglas Hyde, the leader of the communist party in Britain during WWII. Later he renounced his political stand to become a Christian. His book describes how a mere handful of communists (6,000) were able to make a significant impact on the world. He contrasts this with the huge numbers of church members who have made little impact.

The reason for this, Mr. Hyde suggests, is that communists get more from their supporters by asking for more. "He who asks, gets. He who asks for a lot, gets a lot." New communists aren't coddled and spoon-fed. They're immediately placed on the front line before they even have a complete understanding of the communist party line. Usually they were placed in areas of high visibility. Many were sent to sell the *Daily Worker* on London street corners where they had to fend off detractors, attempt to answer questions, communicate, and, most of all, reveal their identities. Of course, they made mistakes. Interestingly, though, this process served to strengthen the new communist's convictions rather than dissuade them. Ask for a little, get a little. Ask for a lot, get a lot.

Persecution does not automatically mean the cause is right. As I've revealed my chiropractic affiliation and commitment, so too have I been assaulted with the horror stories that sabotage this profession's image.

Turning the tables

Between interruptions from beverage and meal service on a recent cross-country flight, my seat mate explained his recent chiropractic experience. After receiving X-rays and beginning care for a period of time, he was improving, but not as completely as he had hoped. He asked the doctor if there was a way to take new X-rays to see his progress.

Suddenly the tables turned. The rationalizations and excuses normally used by patients to avoid the radiation or cost of X-rays came from the doctor. The doctor's reluctance to document the progress of care made a big impression on my new friend.

Prima-facie evidence

Yet without offering patients this visual evidence of chiropractic's ability to make structural improvements, chiropractic will not be able to sufficiently convince the skeptical or the analytical. Those who want more than a "chiropractic aspirin" or who might be available for long-term reconstructive care cannot be identified or persuaded without more evidence. Without proof of an improved form/function connection, even patients who get great results can easily side with medical X-ray specialists who quickly point out that chiropractic doctors seem to find structural problems in every X-ray. Progressive X-rays or other incontrovertible evidence help discerning patients describe their chiropractic experience on more than symptomatic terms. Otherwise, there's an inclination to endorse chiropractic to their friends with nothing more than a half-hearted, "Well, it worked for me." This continues to relegate chiropractic to its current "bad back doctor" orientation, attracting only the intuitive or the desperate. Changing the world's perception of chiropractic to the cornerstone of a wellness approach to health (repositioning) requires successfully reaching the discerning, the analytical, and those who influence others. It will require more than an intellectual extrapolation from feeling better. It requires proof. The same kind of proof used to justify care at the outset of Initial Intensive Care. If we are to enhance chiropractic's image, dynamic X-ray views of the spine may be as important during the later stages of care as they are during the early diagnostic stages.

Interestingly, doctors I meet who regularly take progressive X-rays and perform post-examinations have successful, low-stress practices that don't require strong-arm management efforts to motivate patients. Post X-rays can be important clinical tools that also serve to motivate patients without hype or pressure. Not only feeling their improvement but *seeing* their improvement can speak louder than words.

Another person I met on the same trip had a negative experience, too. She had been on a cruise and had experienced throat problems. A doctor overheard her describe her condition to a friend and asked if he could help. Thinking he was a medical doctor about to examine her throat, she was taken by surprise when he unexpectedly administered a swift cervical adjustment. After three years she is still angry.

Many of the difficulties and challenges that chiropractic faces are not esoteric or even difficult to understand. Rethink chiropractic and approach patients from their perspective. What are their spoken and unspoken fears, concerns, and biases? If they wait until they can no longer stand the pain before calling for an appointment, what should be said and done to reduce apprehension? What can be done to over-communicate, volunteer answers to questions before they are asked, and clear internal dialogue? How can the delivery of chiropractic care be enhanced to reinforce credibility and expertise by anticipating the most frequently asked questions and supplying well thought-out answers?

My role in contributing to chiropractic is not limited to providing a layman's insight into the profession through articles, seminars, or consulting, just as every C.A.'s and D.C.'s role is not limited to providing administration and therapeutics that improve a patient's well-being. Our roles are to explain chiropractic and influence everyone we come in contact with. If we pull any punches, if we avoid our obligation to champion chiropractic in every way possible, with everyone possible, we deserve the condemnation our detractors are only too quick to supply.

Malpractice?

A patient may or may not see the *Reader's Digest* insert. A patient may or may not know about the Wilk's case. A patient may or may not have a wellness orientation. But one thing is certain. Every office, every doctor, and every staff member has the responsibility and the obligation to do everything possible to change a patient's outlook-physically, emotionally, and experientially—while they are in the controlled environment of your office. Anything less is a missed opportunity bordering on malpractice. ■

REPOSITIONING

Everyone who has heard about the UnCola is familiar with concepts of repositioning. Repositioning isn't some new manipulative technique or esoteric practice management procedure. Repositioning is merely a marketing term that describes the process of recognizing a consumer's perception of your product or service and creating a new and better perception to increase its acceptance or utilization. Understandably, chiropractic is a prime candidate for this process. And for those doctors actively pursuing what is now a mainstream marketing strategy, the clinical rewards are significant.

Regrettably, repositioning is something each individual doctor must do. We can't throw money at state or national associations and make it happen as efficiently as it can in your office. Each doctor must recognize the process and implement it in everyday interactions with patients.

Take inventory

First, the current market position must be objectively determined. What does the general public think about chiropractic? Is chiropractic mainstream? Is chiropractic scientific? When would you consult a chiropractic doctor? When would you discontinue consulting one? And that's just for starters. There's no room for wishful thinking or delusions when taking inventory of the general consumer's attitudes and perceptions of the profession. The question is, what do you do with this information?

borns and children under care, a new precedent is set. This shift is called repositioning.

Doctors and their staff must be repositioned before patients can. Not only must you accept that spinal rehabilitation is possible, you must offer patients proof that this phenomenon of long-term Well Patient Care occurs in your office. Do you have the courage to take post X-rays? Or have you rationalized that structural changes don't occur? Are you using empty X-ray view boxes to show examples of before and after X-rays documenting that your patients get symptomatic results and continue on with wellness care? Do you offer a fee structure that makes Maintenance Care affordable and counters the financial barriers sanctioned by insurance companies? What kind of affirmation are you providing patients who continue beyond insurance coverage? How is a patient's non-symptomatic progress documented in this new Well Patient Care model?

Statistically, retention figures become a way to monitor your success in repositioning patients. But let's face it, not every patient is available to be repositioned. However, those who "get" the repositioning message usually refer others with similar mindsets. And that's how you start getting patient visit averages in the 50s, 60s, and higher.

Repositioning our profession for increased utilization will not come from association mergers, a new gimmick, or a slick public relations campaign. It will happen one office at a time, one patient at a time. ■

THE NEW
PATIENT MENU

How accessible is your office? I don't mean its location or easy-to-remember phone number; how accessible is the doctor? In the Bloomington, Illinois *Survey of McLean County Residents' Perceptions of McLean County Professionals,* Doctors of Chiropractic were rated along with 18 other professionals in over a dozen categories, including trustworthiness, honesty, helpfulness, accountability, professionalism, fees, and accessibility. How accessible were chiropractic doctors? Not even in the top 10.

The Bloomington survey was conducted in October 1990 by college marketing students on behalf of the Bloomington area Chamber of Commerce. At several area shopping malls, students asked over 200 people their perceptions of professionals, from realtors and stockbrokers to chiropractors and medical doctors. Sadly, chiropractic placed 19th out of 19 in a majority of the categories. The only bright spot was accessibility, with chiropractic scoring its highest ranking (at 13th). Apparently, the public sees Doctors of Chiropractic as being more accessible than engineers, pediatricians, and attorneys, but less accessible than hospitals (rated 1st in accessibility), physicians (5th), dentists (6th), and even surgeons (11th).

Call screening

While better than being at the bottom (shared by stockbrokers and architects), accessibility for chiropractic doctors is still woefully poor.

C.A.: "Good morning, Dr. SoAndSo's office, may I help you?"

35

CALLER: "Yes, this is Mary Smith, I'd like to speak with Dr. SoAndSo"

C.A.: "I'm sorry, Dr. SoAndSo is with patients right now; can I take a message?"

Terrified that a salesman might slip through, the staff is well trained to limit access to the doctor, even if the doctor is free to come to the phone. The door slams shut on a potential new patient.

Many new patient phone calls are the culmination of many courageous decisions, usually caused by painful symptoms. This fragile decision can take months, even years, to make, slowly moving the patient towards your front door. It is during this process that the effect of all the stories and negative baggage associated with chiropractic is most readily seen.

In the beginning

Every new patient starts out life oblivious to chiropractic. This isolation and ignorance may exist only in childhood. Yet, at some time, prospective new patients learn of chiropractic, although in North America it often has negative connotations. While the public has a growing dissatisfaction with the addictive drugs and irreversible surgery of the medical approach to health care, the observations of the Bloomington study are sobering if you mistakenly think the utilization of chiropractic is suddenly going to explode with the right *Reader's Digest* insert, celebrity endorsement, super bowl testimonial, or the perfect mall show booth design.

After hearing about chiropractic and dismissing it, time passes. If a perceived need (back pain or some clearly spinal-related condition) appears, there may be a perfunctory exploration of chiropractic. "What is chiropractic?" Asking around, your potential new patient asks others about chiropractic. (If he or she locates one of *your* patients and asks what chiropractic is, how well can your patients describe what goes on in your office?)

"I wonder if chiropractic could help," they ask themselves. Yet their painful symptoms have not yet eclipsed their fear. Their decision to consult your office is delayed further. "Anyway, I remember someone saying that chiropractic can make back problems worse."

Remember, this process is going on right now in the minds of the prospective new patients you'll be seeing next month or in the years to come. They drive by your office, know your current patients, and could easily be helped now, but they must make several more decisions first.

Not desperate enough yet

The internal dialogue continues as their condition slowly deteriorates. Since they've heard chiropractic is expensive and painful, there still isn't any compelling reason for them to consult your office. In fact, their symptoms must worsen just to prompt an exploration of conventional medical solutions first. This decision may or may not reduce their pain. At some point, the aspirin, muscle relaxers, and pain pills no longer help, or the patient becomes reluctant to continue using them. Or surgery is suggested, shocking the patient into seeking alternatives. Desperation forces the procrastinator's hand. "Maybe I should try chiropractic," they decide one day. Do they immediately schedule an appointment? No. There are still more "mini-decisions" to be made.

A moment of truth

"Gee, there are so many chiropractors; which one should I go to?" For the first time they are seriously trying the idea on for size. Yet, the internal dialogue continues. "I wonder if it could help." "What would happen if I came in?" "What would my medical doctor, attorney, boss, friend, or spouse say or think?" Peer pressure rears its ugly head, further delaying the decision, lengthening the recovery period, and making care more expensive. And now, desperate, alone, and hurting, they decide to take a big step and call your office. This phone call has taken years to make, yet the staff screens it with suspicion.

"Dr. SoAndSo is with patients right now..."

Even if the patient hasn't lost interest by the time the doctor or new patient coordinator returns and sets up the new patient appointment, the fear lingers. If the staff isn't aware of the low self-esteem caused by finally embracing a "last-resort-not-approved-what-would-my-friends-say-alternative-health-care provider," they may be inclined to treat this potential new patient in an inappropriate, matter-of-fact way. After all, they know that no one has gotten a stroke in your office. Perhaps this insensitivity contributes to some patients' decision to miss their first appointment.

Point of no return

Most doctors and staff don't realize that crossing the threshold into your office is a huge commitment. Few new patients come in the front door, take one look, and leave, although you might reasonably expect them to after hearing the frightening sounds of your adjusting table drop pieces, children crying as they get adjusted, seeing your 1952 X-ray equipment, or walking past the gyrating torsos of those on your inter-segmental traction tables. No, if patients actually make it into your office, it's a significant accomplishment; take their exploratory phone calls more seriously.

Increase your accessibility and help prospective patients move through this multi-step decision-making process more quickly. Consider creating a menu of no-obligation entry points into your office. Here are some ideas you might want to publicize to your community or let current patients know are available:

Telephone access. Doctors available for radio and TV call-in talk shows help callers in the process of making a decision about beginning chiropractic care. If you're not currently available for the media, you could make yourself available to answer questions by phone, perhaps on Mondays during the lunch hour. No elaborate call-screening, just call up and "Ask Dr. SoAndSo your chiropractic health-related question between 12 and 1 p.m. every Monday." Plan to eat in and attack some paperwork when you're not fielding calls. This no-commitment source of information can help move someone along the path towards making a chiropractic decision.

Mail information. How often are you mailing brochures and articles about particular health complaints to members of your community? Have a staff member collect and organize symptomatic brochures, clippings, articles, and other informative materials. If you haven't created an office brochure, do so! At least create a one-page sheet with pictures (and captions) that describes what happens on a new patient's first visit to your office. Let all your current patients know that you have these information packets available; this way they will have access to the resources they need to help those they wish to refer.

Patient referrals. Patients who are referred to your office are almost always less apprehensive and more compliant. Someone they trust has "vouched" for you. You can facilitate confidence among potential new patients who weren't referred by collecting the names of patients who would be willing to take a few short phone calls from prospective patients to answer their questions. Many of your patients would be honored to help you in this way.

The previous suggestions can be effective in moving patients along in their decision-making process while allowing them to remain anonymous. Providing this unconventional level of access can be extremely attractive to a prospective new patient because it acknowledges their reluctance to make the enormous commitment to enter your office. If prospective new patients are ready, there are additional menu choices that can be offered to move them even closer to a chiropractic commitment:

Office tours. You can invite them to tour your office. Use this opportunity to put patients at ease by selecting a relatively busy time of the day. Let them see that the office is successful and attracts other patients like themselves. An experienced staff member can lead the tour and finish it by showing the prospective new patient an educational videotape and introducing the doctor. Staff members can rave about how wonderful their boss is and more easily empathize with a prospective new patient's concerns.

Complementary consultation. This requires even more of a commitment from the prospective new patient. Complementary consultations are widely practiced and well understood. What hasn't been explored are the doctor's expectations and attitude surrounding the outcome of the consultation. Just as animals can sense fear in an opponent, prospective new patients can sense a doctor's desperation to turn someone into a new patient. Automatically expecting them to "sign up" for care is presumptuous and often counterproductive. Respect them enough to let them reach a decision without pressuring them or using scare tactics.

Accessibility is attractive to patients. It removes the unapproachability that creates distance and mystique. Accessibility improves patient rapport, enhancing the healing process and improving the number and quality of the referrals your office receives. How accessible are you? ■

THE CHIROPRACTIC TROJAN HORSE

There's an unseen partner in the examination room with you and your new patient. This silent partner evaluates your recommendations for long-term care very carefully, advises your new patient on the need for X-rays, and strongly influences the decision to refer others to your office. Your willingness to accommodate this third party by providing quality service at a fair price will significantly affect the short- and long-term relationship you have with your new patient.

How much do you pay?

This unspoken dimension to many patient decisions is your fees. While it is easy to philosophize about the importance of good health, it has a price. And since you receive your chiropractic care without any impact on your monthly budget, it makes it difficult for you to understand a new patient's concerns.

For most practitioners and most new patients, insurance usually figures into the mix. Some suggest that insurance has opened the doors to chiropractic to many who would not have otherwise pursued it. Yet thousands of doctors had thriving practices before insurance acceptance, and will likely thrive when higher deductibles, HMOs, and PPOs reduce the role of insurance in the future. Even if insurance acceptance has "validated" chiropractic in the eyes of the public, third-party payers have become something of a Trojan Horse.

The medical model, equating sickness with obvious symptoms, combined with the myopic vision of the insurance industry, has distorted the duration and cost of chiropractic care. Doctors who associated their self worth with a financial statement have greedily set their fees to the upward reaches of the figure accepted by insurance carriers. Catering to the standards suggested by the short-term vision of the insurance industry turns attention away from patient education and a cultivation of the post-insurance patient. After all, with a seemingly endless supply of low deductible new patients, why bother?

Insurance addicts

The implications of this trend are profound. First, the mindless cultivation of short-term insurance cases has created a generation of "insurance junkies." Addicts rationalize that short-term relief care, with assembly-line paperwork and the financial rewards stemming from the easy-to-document symptomatic improvement, is all patients want. They seem to drop out when their insurance coverage is exhausted anyhow! Continuing care would constitute over-utilization, wouldn't it? Providing rehabilitative care requires education and a different kind of clinical expertise. And who said rehabilitative care is even possible? How can you prove the patient needs it? Or document progress? Moreover, does rehabilitative care even work? It's hard to ignore the fact that the frequent visits and X-rays during Initial Intensive Care are simply more profitable (and affirming) than rehabilitative cases that test the doctor's communication skills. Providing symptomatic relief only becomes a self-fulfilling prophecy.

Besides seemingly relinquishing the length and type of patient care to the dictates of insurance carriers, a financial dependency emerges. The financial futures of thousands of chiropractic doctors are figuratively and literally "in the mail," resting on the tenuous future of an industry on the verge of major turmoil and change. More and more policies are offering higher deductibles in order to lower premiums. Municipalities are having to "self-insure" themselves because liability insurance is too high. Rural medical doctors are limiting their practices to "safer" cases, referring even routine obstetric patients to larger cities miles away because of the escalating cost of malpractice insurance. Significant changes in the insurance industry will affect the stock market, the justice system, and the health care community at large. The sky isn't falling, but prudence suggests a closer look at the long-term implications of an unnecessarily high dependence on insurance, simply "because it's there" or "everybody does it" or it's easy.

Ignoring reality

After building a practice and assuming a lifestyle fed on insurance revenues, extricating oneself is difficult, but not impossible. For many, apathy sets in. It's like the American automobile manufacturing executive driving his American-built car to his Detroit office in 1973. Looking out every window as he drives to work he sees nothing but other American-built cars driven by other American automobile executives. And he says to himself, "No Japanese car problem here." Yet the Japanese invasion was well underway 2,000 miles away in California.

How do you encourage patients to continue care beyond short-term insurance coverage? How do you offer more then merely a taste of chiropractic? How can you make spinal rehabilitation a financial reality for a growing number of patients who are wellness oriented? How can you disband the escalating overhead of an expensive insurance processing staff? How do you start easing away from an assembly line pain clinic? How do you avoid the stress created by the need for a constant flow of new patients? How can you end the giveaways, expensive advertising, and other non-therapeutic distractions needed to sustain an insurance-based practice?

Perhaps you first need to recognize that not everyone is available for wellness care. But there may be more patients than you think who merely get lost in the critical transition between insurance and cash. There aren't a lot of good answers to wrong questions, but look at insurance and fees from a patient's perspective.

Avoid misunderstandings

The hocus pocus about fees usually begins on the telephone as patients try to determine how much their care will cost. The automobile

ON BEING
ANTI-MEDICINE

I've met many chiropractic doctors who are actively anti-medicine. Certainly the motive is understandable if you see a constant parade of medical failures and embarrassments enter your office. Yet for the most part, the medical establishment continues to dominate the health care thinking of the general public.

The effects of this distortion are all around us. Television, radio, billboards, even the ads in the magazines of many chiropractic offices bombard us with "solutions" in the form of a pill for everything from back pain to hair loss. And while we know the fallacy of this approach to health, it takes most new chiropractic patients by surprise when they hear their chiropractic doctor get on a soap box and begin M.D. bashing.

Offices most successful in helping patients integrate chiropractic into their lifestyle recognize the following situations or attitudinal patterns created by the medical establishment and develop strategies to effectively deal with them non-judgmentally:

Treatment on the first visit. The book *Bedside Manners, The Troubled History of Doctors and Patients* by Edward Shorter contains the observation that today's health care consumer often consults their medical doctor simply in order to get access to increasingly more powerful drugs. More and more pharmaceutical companies are marketing their wares directly to the general public so patients can tell their doctors which ones they want. When venturing in to see a chiropractic doctor they expect the same degree of relief as that afforded by the first ingestion of medicine. Yet, adjust without taking the time for a thorough examination and report, and you run the risk of devaluing your clinical skills. Adjust on the second or third visit, and the patient may give up on you or become angry before you get the chance. Instead, consider creating an acute new patient routine that allows you to do an exam, educate, give a "mini-report," and treat on the first visit. Use video to educate the patient while the X-rays are being processed and you're seeing other patients. Give a brief report to assure the patient you have a clear understanding of their problem. Then explain and deliver the adjustment and you've fulfilled the patient's expectations without compromising your clinical credibility. Give a complete report of findings on the next visit.

Multiple visits. Since patients seldom get a prescription for a single pill, returning three times a week or more seems plausible at first. But pills seldom cost $25 each! Yes, insurance can help soften the financial blow, however this pill/visit analogy gets chiropractic doctors into trouble as symptoms improve. Get beyond the often unspoken pill/visit metaphor used by most patients to justify visit compliance and begin to explore the idea of "orthodontic chiropractic" or "muscle repatterning" instead. These metaphors transcend the presence of symptoms.

Reception room wait. M.D.s have taught the public to expect to wait and wait, making it the most frequently mentioned irritant among patients. While this would seem to give chiropractic doctors liberty to subject patients to waiting, the reverse is true because of the multiple visits expected by a chiropractic doctor. A survey of patients suggests that 15 minutes is about the maximum allowable wait. Do you know exactly how long your patients are waiting during the 5:30 p.m. rush?

Doctor on a pedestal. More of today's patients have a college education than at any other time in history. Failing to adequately volunteer the hows and whys of his or her recommendations, many medical doctors still hold to the holier-than-thou approach to patient relations. It is hard to tell whether this stems from the outdated notion that patients don't care or wouldn't understand a doctor's explanation. This condescending attitude makes most patients angry enough to increasingly seek second opinions. Active listening is a useful strategy. Ask more open-ended questions instead of a machine gun series of questions requiring only a yes or a no.

Language. Medical doctors have assumed the name "doctors" and chiropractic doctors have been left with the name chiropractors. This reinforces the misconception that chiropractors aren't real doctors. First, always question anyone who uses the term doctor. "Do you mean doctor of medicine or a doctor of chiropractic? There are many types of doctors." Second, when signing your name always use the "Dr." prefix. Yes, it is redundant and maybe even grammatically incorrect when you must also follow your name with a "D.C." The key to any rule is to know when to break it. This is one of those times.

Cleanliness. The medical profession has a name for it: hospital corners. Hospital corners mean your carpet is cleaned right up to the crevice where the walls meet the floor. It's a standard established by the germ theory doctors and the same one chiropractic must meet, even though there is a difference of philosophy. Cologne or perfume on your hands from the previous patient or a dirty chiropractic office immediately causes the patient to question the doctor's cleanliness, attention to detail, and clinical skills.

Afraid to ask questions. Patients have been taught that the doctor's time is precious, so questions are discouraged. This has forced patients to turn to the nurse, pharmacist, or office assistant to ask questions. Same in chiropractic. Which is just one reason why every C.A. should have a working knowledge of anatomy and physiology and understand the terminology used in chiropractic. And it's not always that patients perceive the doctor as being too busy to bother; its a way of getting a second opinion. Patients expect the "party line" from the doctor, but what does a *real* person think about this or that? (Make sure your staff understands that they will need malpractice insurance if they are tempted to cross the line and diagnose!)

Health is passive. Taking a pill to restore "health" turns health restoration and maintenance into a passive undertaking. This attitude can be carried into the chiropractic environment as treatment becomes something that simply happens to a patient, with the responsibility on the doctor's shoulders not the patient's. This active/passive attitude determines a patient's level of compliance and is not changed by recall programs, ambitious computer-generated letter campaigns, or wishful thinking. Chiropractic doctors must educate patients and explain the partnership approach required for maximum results.

Spinal care class. Ever hear of medical doctors asking patients to attend a short talk on the benefits of a particular antibiotic or anti-depressant? While there is growing interest in patient education in the medical arena, it is viewed as an expensive luxury or a way to avoid questions and compliance problems. No wonder there is patient resistance to missing an hour of prime-time television to attend an evening spinal care class. Explain how patients benefit by attending the program (get well faster, save money, prevent the problem from returning, a way spouse can help you, etc.).

Specialty. Medicine has become increasingly more specialized. Fewer and fewer medical students are becoming general practitioners, instead succumbing to the allure (and money) of being specialists. This approach has run wild, resulting in countless medical research projects uncovering detailed information about narrow aspects of human health, virtually ignoring the interrelationship of the studied organ or tissue with other organs and tissues. So while we've proudly heralded chiropractic as the only licensed health care profession expressly dedicated to the elimination and prevention of the Vertebral Subluxation Complex, we've inadvertently become specialists in bad backs. We must always attempt to increase each patient's perception of chiropractic to include a more holistic look at health, with an understanding of the nervous system and not just the local symptoms at the spine.

Payment. A frequent myth held by many doctors of chiropractic is that asking and expecting payment for their services will cause patients not to come back. The reverse is more likely. Call any medical doctor as a new patient and you will be told boldly, without asking, that the initial consultation is $50 (or whatever). Medical doctors have already set the precedent that you pay as you go. Patients look to the implementation of your office policy for clues about your expectations.

Discontinue use when symptoms improve. This is the toughest of all. Written on the side of many over-the-counter medications, this single sentence has done more to perpetuate the myth that you're healthy when the symptoms are gone than all the "Marcus Welby, M.D." episodes combined. This sickness care approach to health has resulted in a generation of patients suffering from diseases that don't have recognizable symptoms until the problem becomes so advanced as to be deadly (cancer and arteriosclerosis), or simply lurks in the background unobserved (hypertension and cholesterol).

Being anti-medicine flies in the face of most patients' personal experiences. While they may be seeking chiropractic care because of ineffective medical treatment, they have had an entire lifetime of what they believe to have been medical "successes." From their perspective chemotherapy, tonsillectomies, antibiotics, polio vaccines, and even temporary headache relief from aspirin affirm that medicine "works." When you're anti-medicine, you take a posture that contradicts most patients' experience and puts your chiropractic recommendations in question.

You can't win by being against medicine. You can only win by being *for* chiropractic. The "enemy" is not the medical doctor down the street, but the health attitudes of the patients who seek your help. If you can successfully "adjust" their attitudes through patient education and a positive chiropractic experience on every level in your office, you'll win. Otherwise, what their medical doctor told them was right. ■

51

doctor, patients make their first tentative phone call, suffering from a type of schizophrenia. They want help, they think chiropractic might help, but they've heard the rumors, the horror stories and so wringing their hands, they make that first call. I believe this mind-set is the rule, not the exception, no matter how well patients cover up their fears or misgivings. It's a new experience. And they're anxious.

The greeting they receive from the staff starts a dialogue that should be sensitive to and accommodate the "pre-existing condition" (medical model health attitude) that exists in the patient's mind.

This puts chiropractic in the same position as the disfigured invalid. Think back to a time when you met someone who was physically disabled or disfigured. Do we say something? Do we try to pretend they're not in a wheelchair? Do we act as if everything is normal? In these situations we look to the disabled or disfigured person for clues about how we should act. Those who recognize their challenge, joke about it, or indicate that they know that we know, and create a climate in which we can put down our guard and be more relaxed and open in our relationship. This is the opportunity faced by chiropractic. Don't apologize, but acknowledge in subtle ways that you know they know by being sensitive to and anticipating the "health care baggage" patients bring to your office.

Besides the obvious questions about high fees, expensive X-rays and the misunderstood need for lifetime care, many new patients think chiropractors aren't real doctors. Here are some other often overlooked misconceptions and attitudes:

First visit treatment. Conditioned by office calls made to the medical profession, patients expect to receive some type of immediate satisfaction, or at least some movement towards relief. You're between a rock and a hard place. Adjust without a thorough examination and carefully designed treatment plan and you devalue your clinical skills. Delay adjusting the patient and the typical patient can become angry, disappointed, suspicious, or all three.

Action step: Validate the care you deliver by describing the amount of thought and clinical experience behind your recommendations and care program. Consider making your new patient process a two-visit procedure. Even if you can size up a case in minutes, resist the temptation for the sake of the patient's perception of chiropractic. Maybe have them return two or three hours later for their first adjustment.

Treatment is going to hurt. The number of patients who tell of being hurt by "other" chiropractors (maybe you!) is almost legendary. Patients are afraid you're going to move the bones too much, twist their head off, or break their back. For those especially fearful, it can become a self-fulfilling prophecy. Regardless of the cause, the result is a major public relations problem. Like bad breath, the patient isn't likely to tell you it has happened unless you convince them you want to know.

Action step: Explain what an adjustment is, what happens, and the importance of total relaxation during the adjustment so you're not fighting each other. This is a wonderful metaphor for the participative, teamwork needed. You both have a job to do–they give you access to their spine by not tensing up, and you apply the smallest amount of non-traumatic force necessary to restore normal motion and position. Let them know how many thousands of adjustments you've given and that you move the bones "just the right amount."

Treatment is risky. "I'm not going to let a stranger get in there and move my bones around," he says almost belligerently, "especially a chiropractor." Or right before a cervical adjustment the patient offers the play-by-play commentary, "And now the paralyzing one." These are defense mechanisms that reveal a lack of patient education or trust. The adjustment should be aborted until the patient's attitude is "adjusted" through dialogue.

Action step: Before the adjustment, use the X-ray findings to show the projected direction and effect of the adjustment thrust. Demonstrate the thoughtfulness you've given it. Explain how many times you've administered this particular type of adjustment since being in practice. Patients need to know that the type of care they are about to receive is personalized, yet routine.

A chiropractor is a "bad back" doctor. Walk into most chiropractic offices and on every wall you will find a display, poster, or model of some form of spinal anatomy. Some offices look like a paleontologist's museum. No wonder patients think chiropractors are bad back doctors!

Action step: Know when "educational" posters are taking the place of some other form of wall accessory. How often are you actually referring to the poster showing the spinal anatomy of a whiplash case? And what is it telling other patients? You seldom see medical doctors with colorful posters touting the medicine they prescribe or the digestive process that sends the drug through the body! The key to changing health attitudes, which is your major competitor (not the medical doctor down the street), should focus on the brain, not the spine. And the most effective way to adjust the brain is through the eyes and ears. Communicate.

The patient is skeptical. Skeptical patients are almost a chiropractic cliche. Even patients who have experienced wonderful results find it difficult to be enthusiastic when telling others, admitting, "Chiropractic probably isn't for everybody, but it worked for me." That helps justify their seemingly bad judgment for having consulted a chiropractic doctor, and takes them off the hook so they don't have to defend their decision. Or what about the patient who told me that when he goes to his chiropractic office he wants to "park in back and wear a sack over my head so no one will see me."

Action step: Accept that every patient over the age of 18 *is* skeptical, especially if they don't refer. On one of their visits, ask what they think makes most people skeptical about chiropractic. Let them answer and agree with them, regardless of how hair-brained their answer is. After they leave, write their response on their treatment card. If you want to increase referrals from this patient, you must successfully put their skepticism to rest, and the only way to overcome skepticism is by offering proof. On subsequent visits you can mention, almost in passing, that you want them to see a new study or read an excerpt of a short article or take a look at some pre- and post-X-rays, or whatever type of proof seems appropriate for their particular type of skepticism. Brainstorm with your staff the types of skepticism and ideas for useful proof. They may be skeptical, too.

The patient feels vulnerable. To top off the skepticism and worries about getting hurt, patients must confess all kinds of health and lifestyle-related information. This exposure, along with the fear of being told that surgery may be necessary after all or they might never be able to live pain free again, is still another source of anxiety. This "white coat syndrome" is also what's responsible for elevating a patient's blood pressure reading 20 points.

Action step: Avoid patients' feeling disoriented by reducing the number of surprises they encounter. Reassure them that nothing will be done without first their complete understanding and agreement. Simplify paperwork, removing references to health-related problems that might be embarrassing, and ask about those in the privacy of the examination room.

The first impression is the most lasting one. And once it's formed, it's difficult to change. Just ask Leonard Nimoy, Vincent Price, Doris Day, or any one who has been typecast after an especially visible success early in their career. Getting new patients through the front door is the easy part. Then the responsibility of changing their perception of health, chiropractic, and themselves begins. When you're successful, you've changed the world in a most important way. ■

MANAGEMENT BY ANTICIPATION

Information, according to those working in the Massachusetts Institute of Technology's Media Lab, is "any difference that makes a difference." Anticipating the future is the surest way to make a difference in it.

The context for doing business changed when we entered the Information Age, yet many businesses still conduct business using an Industrial Age approach, providing tangible commodities to a price-conscious market. Organizations that cling to outdated ways of doing business or fail to anticipate broader customer expectations in the Information Age are likely to experience unexplainable resistance, stagnation, even failure. Price is not everything!

Information packaging

Aside from the effect of the oil shortage of the mid-70s, automobile industry analysts suggest one of the reasons for the successful Japanese invasion was the way the Japanese built, and continue to build, more information into their automobiles. Been in a showroom recently? Detroit is making great strides, but compare dashboards. Do you want to sit in front of an outdated American mechanical contraption or your own jet fighter with digital read-outs? Besides wanting better gas mileage (an intangible), a large portion of the population is choosing the

patients disengage from the office. Then tell them how you'd like them to handle it. Reach a "prenuptial agreement" so you can part friends.

The ability to anticipate is a rare and valuable skill, preventing potential office problems, patient complaints, or situations that interfere with the intangibles of quality, timeliness, or the perceptions of service, attention, organization, and responsiveness. Doctors and staff members with this learned ability improve patient rapport and experience a greater sense of control in their offices and their lives.

By not anticipating the "separation" day, you adopt an emergency lifestyle that increases the feeling of helplessness that often evolves into burnout. Jumping from one brush fire to the next is a stressful way to practice, requiring us to show up at the office with the equivalent of a management suit of armor. A protective suit of steel helps deflect the "slings and arrows" of an unpredictable day. Seemingly uncontrollable circumstances shape the direction of each moment. The day ends with the doctor exhausted, frustrated, and numbed by everyone else's agenda.

The ability to anticipate can be broken into several stages of logical thought. It's the same process, whether you're producing a major patient education video with unpredictable talent or creating a culinary masterpiece for an important dinner party.

Visualize Outcomes. The first step is the most important and overlooked: visualize the outcome you want. Often we enter important interactions with an unusually high level of spontaneity; we become bystanders to the outcome, inventing what we want, believe in, or will support, in real time. Moreover, we often get trapped into the status quo, easily describing what we don't want, but giving little thought to what we'd like to specifically replace it with. The result of this oversight is a string of negatively-worded desires, "I want less stress," or "I don't want to get behind." What do you want instead of less stress? What would be less stressful? The first step is to articulate, in detail and in positive terms, the ideal scenario you want. In this example, what we might want is a smooth-running office in which patients feel they are well cared for and only wait X number of minutes or less.

Devise a Plan. Next, devise a plan to accomplish your outcome. A plan consists of two components: resources and time. The frustration comes from ignoring the finite limits imposed by both–the time it takes to implement specific procedures or techniques and the limitations imposed by office space, layout, the number of doctors, and other resources.

Identify Contingencies. Then, identify every possible failure in the execution of your plan. In advance of your "performance" at 5:30 p.m., list every possible contingency. Cancellations, new patients, and last-minute emergencies are obvious, but what about other influences? Weather, telephone problems, talkative patients, crying children, missing staff members, etc. Use a staff meeting to brainstorm possible response scenarios and solicit ideas from those not directly in the line of fire. They will be less likely to fall into the "we've-always-done-like-this" mind-set and new solutions can emerge. Maybe you've reached your maximum capacity during peak hours, necessitating strategies to increase off-peak volume.

Anticipating patients' needs during the different phases of their care is a crucial skill that builds trust, and, along with active listening, is a fundamental way to demonstrate a "we care" attitude. It is a way to recover control of our destiny in the pursuit of the most honorable calling of all–serving others. ■

MAKING CHIROPRACTIC VALUABLE

Can you remember what it was like not to be able to walk? Not that you couldn't walk, but you didn't know how to walk. It's virtually impossible. Once you know something or experience something, it's difficult to fully appreciate what it was like before you experienced it. Information changes us. It is the result of the information learned from years of chiropractic college that prompts doctors to maintain some type of ongoing non-symptomatic chiropractic care themselves. And it is often this lack of a chiropractic education that accounts for patients' discontinuing care as soon as symptomatic relief occurs.

Your day-in, day-out familiarity with chiropractic can actually create a barrier to patients' getting the necessary understanding and appreciation of chiropractic. Your "expertness" can distance you from "beginners" just starting care. The more you know about something, the more difficult it becomes to communicate it to someone who knows very little.

A computer beginner

I recently purchased a new laser printer for my computer. I hooked it up and it didn't work. I called a programmer I know who works for a large computer manufacturer in our town. "Hey, Rick, how do I get this thing to work?"

"Well, are you using the X-on X-off RS-232 serial protocol or the 8-bit LPT1 parallel interface?"

"Gee, thanks Rick, you've been a big help."

Rick was unable to help me. Ultimately, I had to find a computer "translator" who could. Practically every industry has a technical side to it. A special vocabulary develops that shrouds some pretty basic stuff from outsiders. Maybe some of it is done purposely, although, most of it is created out of expediency or with the honest intentions of saving time or reducing misunderstandings among professionals.

In chiropractic, patients hear terms like subluxation, deductible, MMI, IME, MRI, PI, herniation, spasm, chronic, comp, edema, and the list goes on. These are words and acronyms that doctors and staff use that often insulate patients from understanding and being involved in their care.

Buying patient involvement

This interferes with your ability to motivate and inspire patients. The currency used to purchase patient interest and involvement is information—information that is relevant to the individual patient and presented clearly and volunteered systematically. Clearly, so patients understand. Volunteered, so you don't lower patients' self-esteem by making them have to ask about terms you use so casually. Systematically, so you know what your patients have been told about chiropractic, and specifically their case.

To ensure that the information you share is relevant to the patient, you need to know the patient's wants and needs. It's easy to get carried away and give patients what they need, only to be disappointed later when you discover the patient *wanted* something else. In the same way the doctor's intentions and prognosis can be hidden behind big words, the patients' desires and expectations are hidden in their underlying values and attitudes.

It is the doctor's responsibility to be the "translator," explaining the big words and helping the patient reveal his or her values and expectations. Until the doctor knows what the patient's expectations are, meeting and exceeding them (creating positive word of mouth) is a hit or miss proposition. The process of uncovering a patient's values begins on the first visit, starting with your new patient admitting form.

Succumbing to the obvious, some offices come right out and confront the new, usually hurting patient, asking whether they want only relief care, relief and rehabilitation, or relief, rehabilitation, and prevention. Besides the fact that many patients don't fully understand the ramifications of these concepts, their discomfort on the first visit can distort their personality and their goals. Plus, having heard that once you start chiropractic you have to go for the rest of your life, patients can be reluctant to offer more than a wait and see answer. Instead, take their health attitude pulse more easily (and perhaps more accurately) by asking two additional questions on your new patient admitting form:

How often do you wear seat belts when you drive? Always, sometimes, never (Circle one)

How often do you floss your teeth? Daily, weekly, monthly, rarely, never (Circle one)

Answers to these questions are less likely to be distorted by their current situation and are barometers of their preventive attitudes in other areas of their life. You'll have a better idea what your new patient wants. Don't expect to grow too many maintenance care patients from those who never wear seat belts or floss their teeth!

This observation is based on the idea that you must first reach patients where they are before you can take them to a chiropractic lifestyle. Overnight conversions don't have the staying power of slow, deliberate, step-by-step, growth.

Making chiropractic sexy

Why not ask how often they exercise? Certainly it's worth asking, yet it doesn't necessarily reflect their health attitude. Patients who regularly work out are often people who either want to look better or feel better. Don't confuse someone with a health club membership with someone who necessarily wants to be healthy! Optimum health is not always the primary objective of a regular workout. A newspaper article titled "Sex appeal ranks higher than health" sums up a Florida University study on this topic. ("Sex appeal ranks higher than health," by Anne V.

Hull, St. Petersburg Times, reprinted in the Colorado Springs Gazette Telegraph, January 12, 1991, Page D-4.) Seems that researchers were having difficulty getting patients to lose weight by explaining how unhealthy it is. Instead, they found participants much more interested in dropping the weight at the beginning of a new romance or when motivated by the desire to enhance their sex life. A lowered risk of heart disease and improved overall health and well-being wasn't a big enough carrot. By the way, how are you making spinal hygiene sexy?

Those who provide health care are often shocked to discover that regaining and keeping excellent health is not among everyone's highest priorities. Many chiropractors and their staffs make conscious efforts to live healthy lives and set an example for patients. That's good. Yet, all too often offering bottled water, shunning coffee, crusading against cigarette smoking, expressing shock at vaccinations, and holding up our own lifestyles as examples are counter-productive. Usually this holier-than-thou (healthier-than-thou) attitude rarely makes patients feel uncomfortable enough to rethink the priority they give their health. Anyone who has lowered their credibility by using scare tactics to induce patients to change their ways has been similarly frustrated by a lack of success.

What do patients want?

How do you encourage patients to integrate chiropractic care into their lifestyles and assume a preventive approach to their health? Connect good health with something they value more than their health. It sounds obvious, but if their goal is to feel better, what makes feeling better important to them? Feeling better is rarely an end in itself. Patients often want to feel better for some other reason(s).

If you don't know why each of your patients wants to feel better, you're overlooking an important aspect of the case history. It provides information needed to help patients get what they want, motivate them to do their exercises, modify their lifestyles, follow your recommendations, and continue care beyond just feeling better.

At the conclusion of your examination, when you believe the patient represents a chiropractic case, ask each new patient something like,

"Mrs. Jones I believe yours is a chiropractic case and we've helped many others just like you. I always ask my patients what they hope to do better or enjoy more after they regain their health. Why are you interested in better health?"

Patients aren't accustomed to being asked a question like this. If they're desperate to just "make the pain go away," you may need to help them identify specific activities or dimensions of their lives they hope to enjoy when they are pain free. Are they hoping to improve their golf game? Do they want to be able to pick up their grandchildren pain free? Sleep through the night? What are the key values they find important?

Hole in one

With this information, you have a powerful lever you can connect to their chiropractic care. "So, how's that golf game coming?" you ask on the 5th visit. "Lie down here so we can trim a few more strokes off your game," you say on the 10th visit. Virtually every visit becomes an opportunity to discuss chiropractic and its relationship to the patient's important activity or key motivating value. This association helps patients more easily integrate their chiropractic care into their lives. Maybe that lowers chiropractic in your eyes, but it will probably raise it in the eyes of your patients.

Rarely are patients living to be adjusted. Most are getting adjusted so they can go live. When you find out what your patients are living for, you can increase their desire to follow your recommendations and make chiropractic part of their lifestyle. Become the translator between what your patients want and the chiropractic care they need. When you do, you'll uncover their values and the opportunity to make chiropractic a more valuable part of their life. ∎

BOOMER
BUSINESS

This is difficult to write because I'm a member of the baby boom generation. And like every generation, we have our own idealism, our own foibles, and our own hope for a better future—for ourselves and the world. We are a generation ready, willing, and available for the chiropractic message.

What are you doing to appeal to the unique perspective of this generation?

Born between 1946 and 1964, the baby boom generation is the single largest market segment in the United States. And while we share somewhat similar values and perspectives, there is diversity too. Within this diversity that transcends the work ethic, appearance, and our outlook on life and living is an attitude about health care that should bring joy to every doctor of chiropractic.

Look at the trends reflecting this segment of the population. Hospital occupancy rates are down (in Colorado, they recently averaged only 54% and slipping). Hospitals have to advertise their services and compete by providing seminars and educational opportunities—everything from stress management to "natural" childbirth. Aerobic videotape programs are selling better than many blockbuster Hollywood movies. Diet and specialty cookbooks are on the *New York Times* bestseller list. Alcohol and tobacco consumption are on the decline. High-priced jogging shoes are being designed by aerospace engineers and purchased by ever-discriminating and informed connoisseurs.

There's a decrease in the demand for beef and an increase for poultry, fish, and pasta. There's been a shift in our society.

Times are changing and the baby boom generation, wielding its considerable financial power, has taken a leadership position in making these changes increasingly mainstream.

More and more want prevention

This generation, with its health consciousness, is forcing changes upon virtually every aspect of the health care delivery system. Second and third opinions are more the rule than the exception. House calls? In the December 1, 1986 issue of *Business Week*, a survey among medical doctors shows a significant increase in the number of doctors reviving the custom of making house calls! Moreover, these same M.D.s "expect new patients to shop around for someone whose attitude on health care matches their own." And while many may have a difficult time matching their sickness care approach to health, there's a glut of medical doctors–forcing the need to provide the services today's patient wants. And many want prevention.

Prevention/wellness is a common denominator in this shift in health attitudes. More and more people are making changes in their diets and sedentary lifestyles to embrace preventive measures. Many know their cholesterol count, percent of body fat, and resting heart rate!

How does a "bad back" doctor fit into this new awareness and preventive mind-set? Obviously, without a mind shift on the part of the doctor, this huge market is unaware of one of chiropractic's strong suits: prevention.

The prevention message, when communicated effectively, results in higher retention figures and a lowering of your patient's average age. As patients learn of the preventive aspects of chiropractic, specifically the role chiropractic plays in interrupting (or reversing) the process of Subluxation Degeneration, the demographics change from the 40 to 50 year old with chronic back pain, to the 33-year-old baby boomer bringing in his family. I've seen this shift happen in many offices. None of these doctors have any desire to return to the "pain relief only" good old days.

But concern about one's health is not the driving force among baby boomers. This preventive attitude is a refreshing shift, but I think it's based on a more fundamental aspect: quality.

Patients want quality

We hear it in phrases like, "quality of life," "quality circles," and "quality time." The baby boom generation is unusually sensitive to the subtle qualities that distinguish products and services. Magazines like *Consumer's Reports* pander to this interest. Movie reviewers have their own television shows. Until only recently, American-manufactured automobiles had been shunned by a marketplace casting its vote against planned obsolescence and superficial design changes that are either unsafe, expensive to fuel, or both. Today's discriminating buyer wants quality. At any price.

Voting with their feet

Quality issues are no less a factor within service industries, especially an intangible service like chiropractic. An intangible service is one whose qualities cannot be accurately judged until the moment of consumption. This is not unlike the position the new chiropractic patient finds himself in when beginning care. In Theodore Levitt's insightful book *The Marketing Imagination,* this quality issue, faced by all service organizations, is put into perspective. He suggests that it is crucial that symbols and allusions to the quality likely to be experienced precede the actual delivery of the intangible service. For a doctor of chiropractic that puts a new importance on the quality of business cards. Telephone manners. Office location. Office signage. The reception room. The type and condition of the reception room reading materials. The very smallest of details. (Even the brand name of the VCR you use to play your patient education videos!) And because you and the staff have become accustomed to these symbols, living with them day in and day out, you take them for granted. It makes it difficult for you to see the ragged edges and the less-than-optimal message they may be communicating. These symbols represent the quality of the therapeutics you'll be delivering to a new patient. Symbols that could stand in the way of compliance ("I don't believe you"), or trust ("If you're so good, why is the reception room so shabby?"), and referrals ("I'd be embarrassed to tell anyone I came here."). You'll seldom hear a patient actually say these things. But their actions speak louder than words. They simply vote with their feet.

Using a mirror

There's more to the baby boom generation than preventive health care attitudes and a "white glove" approach to quality. It's their educational background, too. Prompted by parents who wanted their children to "have it better than we did," the baby boom generation is the most educated ever. This educational achievement (25% have college degrees) has reduced the automatic credibility previously afforded doctors, lawyers, and other professionals. No longer is the "do as I say, not as I do" philosophy as effective as it once was. No longer are "doctor's orders" followed automatically and unquestioningly. Today, doctors who experience reduced patient compliance, but who are still smoking, are 20 pounds overweight, or look like the bearded philosophers of a previous century, might discover the diagnostic value of a mirror.

Your staff is probably composed of members of the baby boom generation too. As you might expect, this generation has some pretty clear ideas about work. In 1983, the Public Agenda Foundation conducted a study to determine the top ten qualities people want in a job:

1. To work with people who treat them with respect.
2. Interesting work.
3. Recognition for doing a good job.
4. A chance to develop one's skills.
5. To work for people who listen if you have ideas about how to do things better.
6. A chance to think for themselves rather than just carry out instructions.
7. Seeing the results of their work.
8. Working for efficient managers.
9. A job that is not too easy.
10. Being well-informed about what is going on.

Notice that huge salaries, long vacations, and benefit packages didn't even make the top ten! Ironically, these ten preferences are the very same qualities needed by any business to prosper in the Information Age. Increasingly, baby boomers are looking for career opportunities that foster personal growth, are fun to do (because of constant growth), and reflect their own value systems. They are looking for opportunities to "invest their human capital" in organizations that reflect their values.

Certainly not every aspect of the baby boom generation is admirable. Yuppies are accused of lacking spiritual values beyond consumerism and instant gratification. Yet, the baby boom generation exerts a powerful force in the marketplace. And to practitioners eager to stop "selling" chiropractic to skeptics unwilling to stay under care long enough for real results, the baby boom generation, with its interest in prevention, represents a refreshing new market for chiropractic. ∎

THE THREE PHASES OF STAFF DEVELOPMENT

At what stage of development is each of your staff members? Are you doing and saying the right things to nurture loyalty and commitment? Are you unknowingly sabotaging their desire for a career and setting the stage for high staff turnover?

Calculate the financial and emotional cost of replacing a staff member. Consider the disruption and reduction in your capacity. Try to measure the effect on patients who perceive a lack of managerial prowess. "What happened to Barbara? I was just starting to get to know her..."

Directing the actions of others is just one of the critical managerial responsibilities of running a business. While many doctors yearn for an arrangement where they only have to focus on the healing dimension of chiropractic, staff management will always be part of the daily routine, even with an office manager to assume some of these duties. Success lies in recognizing the changing needs of your staff and systematizing your response so it isn't a continual source of stress.

Much exists to help select and hire new staff members, yet few resources exist for doctors who are thankfully enjoying their third or fifth anniversary with their carefully chosen front desk assistant or X-ray technician. How do you prevent burnout? How do you keep enthusiasm up? How do you avoid losing someone because there is little chance for upward mobility in a small, closely-held business?

First, recognize that given the chance, staff members pass through three stages of development. These stages are not unlike the three stages of care patients experience. Like patients, some are not available for anything more than a job (Initial Intensive Care). Some continue with Rehabilitative Care and discover a career (Maintenance Care).

Encourage continued growth

Why do some patients fully integrate chiropractic into their lifestyle, while others remain hopelessly unavailable? While it doesn't guarantee longevity, patient education plays an important role in this process. Use this same sensitivity to create and nurture a loyal and committed staff by changing your "management" strategy during the three phases of employment: Entry, Excitement, and Empowerment. These three phases acknowledge that people remain in situations where they are growing, and leave situations when they stop growing.

The Entry Phase. The Entry Phase covers the hiring process and about the first month or so in the office. Offices interested in creating lasting staff relationships test applicants not only for necessary skills (typing, math, filing, etc.) but also for a shared value system. Because even if a potential new staff member can file flawlessly and type 100 words a minute without error, if there isn't a shared value system and pre-existing "health awareness," you are looking at a short-term relationship. It will never be more than a job.

How do you test for values compatibility and health awareness? First, ask what's important to them. Have them think of someone they used to work with. What were some of the values or characteristics of that individual they especially appreciated? What are some of the important values they want others they work with to have?

Interviewing for a sense of health awareness is somewhat difficult, since you will probably be dealing with candidates weaned on the medical model. Don't let that distract you! What you're looking for are people in touch with their own bodies who will have a better chance of empathizing with patients. Again, give them a chance to reveal their health attitudes while talking about someone else. Have them think about someone they know who they perceive as being very healthy.

Then have them describe some of the characteristics that contribute to that person's health. Then reverse the question. Have them think about someone who isn't healthy and describe those characteristics. You're not looking for clinical insights; you're looking for their use of language, sensitivity, and other subtle clues. Because many people become self-conscious at job interviews, trying to give the "right" answer, help them feel more comfortable by focusing their attention on someone else.

The rest of the Entry Phase is obvious if you recognize the mind-set of your new staff member: they want to win. So, during their initial phase in the office they are likely to be very "I" directed. How can *I* do the right things? How can *I* not make a mistake? How can *I* look good to my new boss? After a rudimentary explanation of chiropractic, its purpose, and its language, the primary focus should be procedural. Help your new employee feel and look competent as quickly as possible. Chiropractic philosophy falls on deaf ears in the same way new patients cannot hear the key words in your report of findings when they are still in pain.

As soon as the basics are mastered, staff members are available for the Excitement Phase.

Excitement Phase. Because the most pressing need when hiring a new staff member is often clerical in nature, it's easy to neglect the development of the naturally occurring Excitement Phase. Or, before investing too much time and energy in staff education about chiropractic, we decide to wait and see if your new protege will "work out." And they do. They master the clerical side of the job quickly and start looking so good, we forget that their chiropractic knowledge is as superficial as that of most patients entering the practice. And because their chiropractic education is not systematized, getting a staff member truly excited about chiropractic is time-consuming and takes a second place to maintaining patient flow. This is why the Excitement Phase is usually remembered by most new staff members as the Endurance Phase! Without a vision of chiropractic larger than that of the apparent solution to an endless string of patients suffering back problems, being a chiropractic assistant becomes a repetitive job with little fulfillment.

With the mastery of office procedures, your new staff member can look beyond the "me" orientation of the Entry Phase and is available for a "you" perspective. Only now is your staff member available to begin the process of nurturing patients. "How are *you* doing today, Mrs. Jones?" Respond by laying the groundwork for them to have a career in chiropractic. They should be learning everything they can about chiropractic. Spend lunch hours and staff meetings sharing your chiropractic philosophy. Send your staff home with books and audiotapes. Encourage questions. Share the clinical progress of some interesting cases. Get them involved beyond the mere clerical. Remember, you're battling an entire lifetime of health attitudes shaped by the germ theory and the belief that ill-health is only associated with obvious symptoms. Use this time to explain your adjustment technique, X-ray analysis, and the many other things you do. Show your post X-rays. Celebrate your victories. Share your frustrations. The objective is to deepen their involvement beyond keeping a neat appointment book. Remember that patients are seldom more excited about chiropractic than your staff is.

Wait too long before developing this awareness in your staff, and you miss an important window of opportunity that may doom the future of your new employee.

Soon your newly-hired staff member will be ready for the Empowerment Phase.

Empowerment Phase. You'll know when your staff member has entered this stage of development when you discover their new sense of initiative. Now, the sense of "we" emerges. A sense of "psychic ownership" in the practice blossoms.

If lateral moves within the office aren't available, such as becoming a new patient advocate or performing preliminary patient exams, your employee may have exhausted the opportunity for continued professional growth. Seize this opportunity by continuing their growth on a personal level. And while the specifics vary with each individual, help your staff member identify areas of potential self-development. This is when it makes sense to invest in your staff through a Dale Carnegie course, advanced chiropractic seminars, public speaking programs, business communications classes, and a whole range of other activities whose dollars and cents return to the clinic may only be indirect or long term. The strategy here is to maintain some form of growth so your employee remains alert, vibrant, and alive.

Doctors who recognize these changing stages of employment can respond appropriately. Motivating the staff is easier when you can see that the source of job satisfaction changes during the course of employment. It takes extra effort, but it is a small price to pay for reduced turnover, sense of team, and the stability that patients want in an environment designed for healing. ■

THE COST OF OWNERSHIP

A crucial link in having patients fully experience your educational program is an enthusiastic and committed staff. Yet, high staff turnover within chiropractic interferes with this critical procedure. Sadly, staff turnover is so widespread, many doctors accept it or merely shrug it off as the cost of doing business. And it's a very high cost.

The subject comes up in patient focus groups I've held for offices that have experienced high turnover. It's demoralizing for patients to see a new face behind the front desk, and it raises questions about behind-the-scenes working conditions and the doctor's management abilities. It lowers the image of the office and the credibility of the entire staff. As in other businesses with high turnover–fast food restaurants, car washes, or convenience stores–it's expensive, disruptive, and redirects large amounts of energy away from serving your patients.

If you have the wrong people or have harnessed their potential incorrectly, get on with the inevitable! You're doing them, the office, and the future of chiropractic a disservice.

A job versus a career

For many, the selection, hiring, training, and nurturing of staff members is the most challenging aspect of running a chiropractic office. If success has been spotty, it may require a shift in attitude and approach. Without change, your practice and profession stand to be hurt in the future as members of the baby boom generation become fully integrated into the work force. As the number of available workers diminishes, chiropractic will have to face up to salaries that ignore the realities of an increasingly competitive marketplace and training programs that limit staff positions to narrowly-defined, repetitious, task-oriented, burnout-producing jobs.

Pay more?

But is the solution more money, more benefits, and more, more, more? No. No. And no. How do the best-run companies avoid expensive staff turnover and create career positions? Ownership.

Not literal ownership. Not co-signing your bank loan. Not putting their name on the clinic sign. Not a bigger desk in the corner office. Not even a raise. Psychic ownership. A sense of belonging. A real feeling that it's "our" practice. If you have the right staff and you want to keep them, here are some ways to help nurture a sense of psychic ownership in your practice.

Team linguistics

The first involves semantics; how the doctor uses language to describe office activities. Most small business owners work very hard to build their businesses. Almost single-handedly they've kept the bill collectors at bay during the early days. It's their vision and their name on the sign out front. Naturally there's the tendency to call it "my business" or "my practice." If you're interested in remaining the Lone Ranger, stunting the commitment of those around you, continue to call it such. But the most successful business leaders recognize the contributions of their staffs and refer to their business as "our business" or "our practice." It seems such a small thing, but employees are sensitive to it, and swell with pride when they hear it.

A corollary of the my/our practice is the "my girl" reference so often heard in chiropractic circles, as in, "I'll have my insurance girl call you..." Besides being sexist, it's demeaning, it's dictatorial, and it's out of touch with the language that motivates and inspires team support in the 1990s.

Another way to build psychic ownership is to involve the staff more closely in patient care. Doctors are in the enviable position of experiencing a sense of progress with patients. Patients enter the practice almost desperate, and over a period of days, weeks, or months, regain their health. Sure, it's fulfilling. Yet, for the staff insulated from this primary source of inspiration, progress is measured in less satisfying terms: kept appointments, running on time, and other mundane interactions. Staff members can feel a sense of psychic ownership when they are kept up to date on the clinical progress patients experience, feeling a vicarious sense of participation in the caregiving process.

Promoting a sense of psychic ownership requires a sense of team. Building a successful team, whether in sports, politics, or health care, requires these six ingredients:

1. A common purpose. Is there a statement of purpose that everyone understands, supports, and aspires to? Does the staff know the long- and short-range goals of the doctor? Must staff members derive intentions solely by the doctor's behavior, or does the doctor freely communicate office objectives?

2. Appropriate division of labor. Does everyone understand their duties and how they contribute to the intended outcome of the practice? Are job descriptions specific, yet flexible enough to allow growth? Are staff members laterally trained so they can cover other positions in an emergency?

3. Accepted leadership. Even though it's the least glamorous part of running a small business, have you embraced your leadership role, providing management direction? Or do you depend upon a "from the hip" response to the latest emergency? Is your management style participatory or dictatorial? Have you dealt with the differences between being liked and being respected?

4. Agreement on the plan and process. Is there a detailed procedural manual that empowers the staff to make necessary decisions? Or is every new staff member inventing their job? Do staff members constantly have to "check with the doctor" on too many issues?

5. Solid relationships of mutual trust. A good indication of this is whether staff members see other staff members in social, non-working situations. Or does everyone come together during clinic hours just because they have to?

6. Good communications. This may be the most important of all. Are there frequent staff meetings? Proximity does not guarantee communication—or understanding. Is the door always open to talk about any issue? Even the Emperor's Clothes?

Team celebrations

These six issues contribute to the sense of teamwork important to psychic ownership. Another overlooked component in nurturing a sense of psychic ownership is in celebrating together. Often intra-staff communications are limited to problems—with patients, insurance companies, or others. No wonder we avoid staff meetings! Instead of discussing the three negative patients, stress the 10 unusually pleasant or appreciative patients. Have everyone collect and share at least one positive experience they had during the week at each staff meeting. Consider occasional meetings outside the office to give your meetings a fresh outlook and perspective.

The doctor as a coach

Another vital aspect of psychic ownership is the way day-to-day management and supervision take place. When the doctor hovers over the appointment book it undermines confidence and communicates a lack of trust. Reactions to new ideas determine the willingness to volunteer future ideas. How you handle the inevitable mistakes teaches risk taking. How the doctor stands up for staff members in disputes with vendors or others is a barometer of trust and respect. Today's successful manager is a facilitator, cheerleader, and coach.

Providing opportunities for staff members to have psychic ownership takes confidence. Since psychic ownership cannot be purchased with higher paychecks, it is a rare quality. But to bask in its power takes the biggest risk of all. It requires honesty in facing limitations. Exposing hidden agendas to others. Even rejection or allowing others to take advantage of a vulnerability you've extended. But above all, it may require doing the most terrifying thing we ever do: change. ■

THE SECRET OF MOTIVATION

Sometimes it seems the harder you try to get patients to understand the value of a chiropractic lifestyle, the less effective you become. In fact, many offices employ approaches to motivate their staffs and patients that are actually counterproductive, creating an unhealthy, dependent relationship.

Recall programs, the equivalent to a hotel morning wake-up call, are a good example of how doctors assume too much responsibility for their patients. Without a thorough understanding of the nature and severity of their condition, patients naturally can't assume the responsibility to value their health sufficiently to show up for care. It's a matter of motivation. How do you motivate patients to take responsibility?

Since 1986, at seminars around the United States and Canada, I have been intrigued by the topic of motivation. Invariably after a seminar someone will approach me, thanking me for a "motivational" seminar. "I don't remember covering the topic of motivation during the seminar," I say. "On what page of the notes did we discuss motivation?" Of course, talking about motivation doesn't result in motivation. All I do is present ways for doctors and their staffs to get acquainted with new possibilities for their offices. Perhaps they have reached a plateau, are in burnout, or feel trapped, thinking they're stuck in the current version of their office for the rest of their lives. All I did was show them new ways to get involved and become rechallenged. It seems that motivation comes from the new possibilities for involvement in one's life. To care again. To have purpose.

The spoiled child

A classic example of assuming too much responsibility and eliminating opportunities for involvement is the child who has been pampered his entire life and then, by some misfortune, inherits a highly successful business venture or a large sum of money. Isolated from the details of actually running the business, even as an adult, the founder's son quickly squanders the fortune and runs the business into the ground. When we assume too much responsibility for our children, or anyone else, we sabotage normal development and the self-esteem necessary for a healthy, balanced life.

Closer to home, the role involvement plays in the creation of motivation is illustrated by looking at the purchase of a new office photocopier.

The parable of the new copy machine

Let's say your office needs a new photocopier. The old one is frequently jamming and it lacks many of the features newer models offer. The staff has been complaining recently about the machine, and it's time for a new one. The tendency for many doctors with Type A personalities is to march out and buy a copier. Want a copier? Here. Suddenly a new machine shows up one morning, surprising the staff. Instead of jubilation, the staff seems distant and depressed. While the doctor's quick response and willingness to properly equip the staff is admirable, it demotivated them. What happened?

By assuming total control of the copier problem, the doctor eliminated the opportunity for staff involvement. Plus, this new machine (that, ironically, the doctor rarely uses) doesn't have the enlargement and reduction features the staff really wanted. Yes, they got their machine, but in their eyes it's the wrong machine. Plus, they didn't get the pleasure and the affirming sense of "team" by researching, pricing, and testing competitive models. Was it more expedient than involving the staff and wading through all the personalities and concerns? Sure.

But in the process, the staff was demoralized at a time when a purchase like a copy machine could have been a rallying point for improved productivity. Sometimes the process (involving the staff) is as important as the destination (getting the copier).

More delegation!

Fundamentally, this is a delegation problem. It may be a symptom of a lack of trust or just the desire to prevent staff members from failing at a task. Yet, failure is a necessary part of the learning process and taking responsibility for ourselves. Certainly if failure creates a life or death situation, avoidance is important. That's rarely the case. It's usually an expediency question where it would be faster to do it ourselves than to explain it to someone else. When doctors take this tack, they soon find they're doing all kinds of non-clinical activities, stealing responsibility and its resulting motivation from the staff. Learning to delegate is an acquired skill and especially difficult for those with perfectionist tendencies.

Unfortunately, we are all guilty of taking opportunities away from those we work with and stealing their motivation in the process. Staff meetings are good examples. Staff meetings should be organized and run by the staff. After all, that's what they're called: *staff* meetings. Instead, many doctors turn this valuable team-building occasion into a monologue that siphons off the motivation and energy of the staff. Forget the tirades about statistics and telephone procedures, the real signal being sent by the doctor is "this-is-*my*-practice-not-*our*-practice-and-you're-just-employees-here."

Patient motivation by doctor and staff is often sabotaged in similar ways. Here are a few overlooked situations where the intent is usually well-meant, but the result sabotages the patients' ability to get involved and take responsibility for themselves:

Insufficient patient education. "If patients knew what I know they'd become lifetime patients and refer all their friends," wailed a doctor in frustration. And that's true. Since the Vulcan Mind Meld popularized by Mr. Spock on "Star Trek" hasn't been patented yet, a variety of patient education techniques must be used to get the chiropractic message to patients. Without a complete understanding of their problem, and the truth as to how long it will take to bring it under control, patients can judge their progress only by how they feel. If chiropractic care is something that merely "happens" to patients, they are isolated and shut out from being involved. Information is a way you involve and motivate your patients. Jan Carlzon, in his book *Moments of Truth*, observes, "Anyone who is not given information cannot assume responsibility. But anyone who is given information cannot avoid assuming it."

Real time examination test results. Many offices model their examinations after the medical model, asking questions, having patients perform certain actions, taking notes, and "Hmmming" in an all-knowing, doctorly way. But this approach angers patients. Tell me my blood pressure now! Tell me what you're discovering now! Is there hope? I want to know! Many patients are silently begging for a chance to be involved and instead are forced to wait for a "super-duper-it-can't-fail-wait-until-they-hear-this" report of findings. No single report will magically transport patients from a symptom-oriented medical approach to health to a preventive chiropractic lifestyle. Use the examination process as a way to involve patients by foreshadowing the recommendations that will follow at your report of findings.

Report of findings. The report is another occasion where involvement and the resulting potential motivation can be thwarted by assuming too much responsibility for the patient. I've heard a doctor say, "I'm going to take care of those headaches for you" or "Bring your husband in for care and we'll fix his low back pain." Aside from the obvious risk of promising a cure, this style of communication strips patients of their responsibilities, such as keeping appointments, paying their bill, and following recommendations. Try instead, "Together we're going to work on those headaches" and "When your husband is ready, bring him in so we can help him with his low back pain." The health problems patients present when they enter the office are *their* problems, not yours. That doesn't mean you can't be sensitive, compassionate, and caring. But never take away the patients' responsibility for their role in the restoration and maintenance of their health. It's their health and they deserve the right to fail if they wish.

Asking questions. If patients are interested enough in chiropractic and their health, they may be inclined to ask questions. In fact, the number of questions patients ask is a good indicator of their involvement. Yet, if their questions are greeted with a Mr. Know-it-all attitude, questions will stop coming. If patients are still interested, they may ask staff members questions. A question is a most magnificent thing. It reveals so much about the person asking the question—and the person answering it. If patients don't ask questions, you can help keep patients involved in their care by asking *them* questions. "Now why do you suppose your right leg is always short?" or "Why do you suppose that when I do this, you feel it down your arm?" Asking questions can help patients think in new ways and discover themselves through their chiropractic experience.

In the heat of battle, the motive always seems right: to save time, to avoid mistakes, or to prevent a relapse. Frequently these attempts backfire and create dependent relationships. A career for the staff is reduced to a job. And a significant lifestyle change for patients becomes merely a "natural aspirin" to be administered only when symptoms are present. Allow patients to fail gracefully, without judgment. Permit the staff to become more fully involved through delegation. Raise their self-esteem by creating new opportunities to be involved, motivated, and independent. ■

ASKING
QUESTIONS

One of the most frustrating attitudes to deal with in chiropractic is the rejection that comes from indifference, which is the attitude most people have when it comes to the subject of chiropractic. Maybe indifference, with just a hint of suspicious skepticism.

People who are indifferent to chiropractic, or active skeptics, are unlikely to change their minds, even with the most passionate explanation. And while the sparring match may evoke a renewed sense of purpose, confronting the skeptic is usually a waste of time. Sadly, these are the people who garner the most attention and focused concern in many offices. They are the two or three patients who say something to question the validity of chiropractic or a wellness approach to health. They can't be ignored, yet the real excitement is opening the eyes and ears of the indifferent!

You can help transform indifferent patients into champions for chiropractic by "engaging" them. Engagement is capturing someone's attention to communicate the chiropractic message. The rancher who hit his mule with a 2-by-4 to get its attention understood what engagement is all about!

The pain clinic

Pain is the "2-by-4" that initially engages patients, urging them to investigate chiropractic. After attending my first chiropractic seminar in 1981 to research what ultimately became known as the Peter Graves video, I consulted a doctor of chiropractic who had been recommended to me to find out what phase of Subluxation Degeneration my spine was in. Imagine the doctor's shock when I showed up in his "pain clinic" without any symptoms! Every form, every question, and every procedure was oriented for someone suffering from one of the 13 (or is it 14 this week?) warning signs.

Of course you're feeling better

This generation and probably the next, unless more offices make pediatric chiropractic attractive, will seek chiropractic care because of some type of ache or pain. Pain can be a very engaging reason to overcome the fear of the unknown. But as generations of chiropractic doctors already know, the pain usually goes away. And so do the patients. If chiropractic is to become the predominate health care delivery system, relief of pain must be thought of as just one of the several by-products of doing something even more important—stopping, slowing down, or reversing the process of Subluxation Degeneration. Keep in touch with the affirmation that symptomatic improvement affords, but own the idea that it's merely an expected sign post on the higher road of a preventive, wellness approach to health care. If you want to help reposition patients, extending their vision of a doctor of chiropractic beyond a "bad back" doctor, avoid the temptation to rejoice too visibly when patients tell of their newfound symptomatic relief! After all, do you celebrate the light created by turning on a light switch? Do you throw a party every morning when the sun rises? "Of course your symptoms have improved; now we can get to work on an even more exciting aspect of chiropractic—spinal rehabilitation!"

Clearly, without a systematic, ongoing patient education program, a patient's engagement with chiropractic is likely to end prematurely. There are large sums paid to management firms for ideas to re-engage patients, but many are ineffective. Recalls. Reduced fees. Pleading. And the well-meaning but suspicious, "The-doctor-needs-to-see-you-for-one-more-visit" scripts that are interpreted as a desperate move to save a financial resource. It's too late.

If patients must be fully engaged and perceive an appropriate cost/benefit ratio for continued care, how do you accomplish this after the benefits they originally sought have been delivered and their pain is gone?

First, recognize that a portion of the population will not avail themselves of rehabilitative or preventive health care. These are the people who require state mandated automobile inspection programs to detect unsafe mechanical defects in their cars. They refuse to brush their teeth regularly. Or wait to do their laundry until the moment they need a clean shirt. This is a pattern developed early in life and as great as chiropractic is, it's unlikely to overcome the momentum of a myopic lifestyle.

Everyone directly or indirectly connected with the delivery of chiropractic must help each patient remain engaged.

Engaging patients

One way to engage patients to help them internalize their chiropractic experience, and equip them to tell others about chiropractic is to regularly ask them questions. There are three types of questions. The first is the "inquisitive" question. As you would expect, its purpose is to uncover information you don't know. When were you born? How long have you been experiencing this problem? Inquisitive questions give you the basis for making recommendations. Because the information flows one way, relationships based on this type of questioning are very shallow. Think how engaged you are with most salespersons, order takers at restaurants, car mechanics, M.D.s, and others who just ask perfunctory, inquisitive questions. These types of questions are necessary, but limit the level of engagement.

Another type of question is the "surprise" question. Reporters Sam Donaldson and Barbara Walters ask a lot of these. They're used to catch you off guard, upset you, or encourage new ways of thinking. "How come you waited 35 years after falling off your bicycle to come in here?" is a surprise question. It repositions the subject at hand and enhances the creative process. These types of questions can be perceived as confrontational, however, and should be used with caution.

The best type of question to use with your patients on a daily basis is the "supportive" question. The best consultants use these questions when working with their clients. And the best doctors remember to use them regularly with their patients. Supportive questions are questions you ask when you already know the answer! It's a Socratic method of reaching the truth. The answer cannot be provided disinterestedly; the question almost forces engagement.

Supportive questions are often used in courtrooms. Unlike Hollywood's dramatic portrayal, there are few surprises in courtroom testimony. Anyone doing regular PI work recognizes that the court is just a laborious way to expose what is usually already known.

When a consultant discovers a doctor's patient visit average has risen from 30 to 50, he or she knows there are only a few reasons for this increase. So when a good consultant asks, "What do you think accounts for the increase?" it's not because he or she doesn't know the basis for computing this revealing statistic! Something more important is happening. By having to formulate an answer, the doctor becomes engaged, actively participating in the process of diagnosing the practice. When supportive questions become the primary tool in a consulting environment, growth and insights can occur without a dangerous dependency upon the consultant. The same is true with patients. When you enlarge a patient's understanding of his or her health, you create a partner, not a dependent child who must be "managed." Each interaction becomes an exciting growth experience. This teaches self-responsibility and fulfills the doctor's obligation to be foremost a teacher.

When a patient volunteers, "Whatever you're doing, doc, I'm really feeling better," instead of basking in the glory, are you asking the supportive and totally engaging question, "Why do you think that is?"

Total engagement.

Some very important things happen when you remember to capitalize on opportunities to ask patients supportive questions. First, for at least a moment, they are completely focused on their health, searching for the words needed to internalize and describe their chiropractic experience. In a sense, they "practice" explaining their perceptions in front of you so, if needed, you can gently correct any misunderstandings revealed by their answers. When your patients have the chance to share chiropractic with others, they're more likely to be articulate, accurate, and positive in their descriptions.

Patient #1: "Why don't I feel better yet?"

D.C.: "Tell me why you think that is."

Patient #2: "I can't come in next Wednesday."

C.A.: "How do you suppose that will affect the results you want from your chiropractic care?"

Like any tool, asking supportive questions takes practice. It's a powerful way to help patients more fully "own" their chiropractic experience, and also creates better referral ambassadors for chiropractic–and you. ■

FEATURES
AND BENEFITS

"I wish I had more new patients." "It's hard to get patients to attend my spinal care class." "I don't think my yellow-page ad works as well as it should." "I feel like no one's reading our clinic newsletter." "It's hard to get patients to continue care after their insurance coverage ends." "How do I get patients to refer?"

Have I missed any?

We get so immersed in our specialized areas of interest that we forget how to communicate in a language the outside world understands. We forget the simple, compelling, often selfish and motivating reason(s) for which we originally got involved in chiropractic. Or worse, we don't try to communicate, assuming by virtue of a patient's proximity to us or the obvious "rightness" of our beliefs, our language is self-explanatory.

Feeling cocky?

Ask your best patients to describe what you do. "I was just wondering, how do you describe what goes on in our office to your friends and family?" Pay particular attention to the language they use. If you're brave enough to ask, you're likely to hear the verbal equivalent of a child's first attempts on a violin. And you wonder why only a few patients seem to refer others! At least when I get my prescription filled or my dentist fills a cavity, I can easily tell others what happened.

Amazingly, a lot of doctors don't explain even the most basic doctor/patient encounter, so patients can't be articulate when there is an opportunity to tell others about chiropractic. And it's not just explaining chiropractic–it's being able to defend their decision for consulting you!

Yellow-page ads trumpet the 13 warning signs and merely confirm why the prospective patient consulted the chiropractic section in the yellow pages in the first place. If you were looking in the yellow pages for a car mechanic and all you saw was ad after ad with the same list of problems the mechanic fixed, you'd still have very little information on which to base your buying decision.

The lack of patient rapport, inarticulate patients, and inept yellow page advertising overlook today's currency: information. Information is power. And the more information you can convey to current and prospective patients, the more "powerful" you and your patients become.

Making a fast get-away

In a highly relevant book for health care providers, *Service America!* authors, Karl Albrecht and Ron Zemke describe the growing service sector of our economy. The hierarchal General Motors pyramid of the 1950s has been foisted upon unknowing doctors by consultants who think Industrial Age manufacturing models are efficient means to run service organizations of a dozen or fewer employees. This has created two obstacles to practice growth. The first is evidenced by a continuous stream of "I'll have to check with the doctor" by a paralyzed staff. The second is the most destructive. It's the "I'm-just-the-C.A." game. Here the staff has mentally checked out. They've taken on the mentality of an impotent factory worker. They're the ones who back their car into their parking space, ready for a quick get-away when they're unchained and "punch out" at the end of the day.

People commit their energies to the extent that it gets them what they want. Period. For employees, it's not always just money–a paycheck or a bonus. It may be psychological, wanting a sense of completeness or praise. It may be a feeling of teamwork, shared experience, or working in the pursuit of a bigger idea. Until you find out what rewards motivate your staff, staff management is just a stressful and manipulative technique to get them to do things. Same with your patients.

Another way of saying that people commit their energies to the extent that it gets them what they want is that people buy benefits, not features. We write checks, borrow money, or consult a chiropractic doctor because of how it will benefit us. This seems obvious, yet it's often forgotten when communicating with patients. Reread the first paragraph of this chapter. How many of these problems are caused by patient benefits not being clearly explained?

Intangible benefits

The benefits people buy are not always tangible. A Mercedes automobile isn't marketed for its tangible benefits of getting you from point A to point B. The brochure focuses on the intangible benefits. The color of the car is merely a feature. The fact that the car says so much about us is a benefit. The fact that it has leather seats is merely a feature. The way I feel about myself when I smell the leather is a benefit. Some of the most powerful, motivating, and overlooked benefits are intangible.

What are the features and tangible and intangible benefits of the chiropractic care you and your staff provide in your office?

Patients seek out your office because they want some form of relief they've heard chiropractic can offer. Initially, this relief is the primary benefit (source of motivation) a patient experiences. Whether they pay cash, write a check to cover the deductible, or simply show up, they are exchanging their money and time to receive the benefit (as they perceive it) of chiropractic care.

Then they're invited to a spinal care class. As if they should know what a spinal care class is and how it can benefit them! Until you make that vital translation from the spinal care class (feature) to what it would mean to your patients by helping them get well sooner (benefit) or helping them to prevent a relapse (benefit) or save money (benefit), you're wasting your time.

Of course, you could make the class mandatory, discontinuing patients' care unless they attend. This, along with scare tactics and other forms of manipulative patient control methods, is tempting because it may be effective in the short run, yet it sabotages long-term relationships.

Consider the way patients are presented with the opportunity to see patient education videos in the office. The tapes are merely one of the many features of your office. They are no more valuable to a patient than an adjusting table or some other piece of furniture until patients understand the benefits of seeing them. If the staff doesn't perceive the benefits of being armed with the information presented in your patient education videos, they are unable to present the videos with enthusiasm and passion. Consistent, effective implementation is based on identifying the benefits of the program—for both staff and patients.

A feature is merely a characteristic of a product or service. It's big, it comes in 12 colors, it's a technique called Gonstead, it's the fact you have a spinal care class, accept credit cards, or have your office open on Saturdays. They're just features. They have little value unless someone sees how a particular feature can provide a benefit.

Become a translator

A benefit translates a particular feature into human terms. Convenience, prevention, saves money, speeds recovery, reduces pain, prevents the problem from returning, saves time, makes you feel important, etc. Benefits are the red buttons that motivate patients, inspire staff members, and build practices.

Like motivation, the benefits of a patient's chiropractic experience may be intangible. What are the benefits of watching a patient education video? What are the benefits of attending a spinal care class? Or a progressive examination? Or reading your clinic brochure? Or showing up on time? Or paying? Help patients see that they benefit by doing what you want them to do. That's the only form of "control" you ever really have over anyone. Any other form of control is merely a myth.

Without translating clinic policies and daily routines (features) into motivating benefits, the routines needlessly insulate and alienate patients. "Mrs. Jones, I'm reserving Wednesday at 3:15 especially for you so the doctor can devote his total attention to you and your case." "Jerry, I'd like you to review this literature. It will explain how problems just like yours respond to chiropractic care and how you can speed your own recovery." Translate the features of your practice into benefits for the patient. The benefits of getting a 10% discount for paying cash are obvious for most patients. But the benefits of spending an hour in a spinal care class instead of being home with their family may not be.

Make a list

At the next staff meeting, brainstorm the features of your practice. Tangible and intangible. There are lots of them. Then put yourself in your patients' shoes and translate the features into patient benefits.

First, why your office and not someone else's? (Benefits of convenience, accessibility, fees, personality, rapport, confidence, etc.) Why continue chiropractic care beyond symptomatic relief? (Benefits of keeping the problem from returning, continued good health, feeling a sense of progress, etc.) Why find out more about chiropractic through patient education opportunities? (Benefits of being a more articulate spokesperson for chiropractic, participating in health-related decisions, being able to defend the choice you've made to consult a chiropractor, being perceived as someone who knows something, etc.) Why refer others to the office? (Benefits of helping others, being appreciated by the doctor, etc.)

Until you discover the benefits that motivate those around you, life is just an unexplainable series of random events. And taking control of the practice is an unattainable, burnout-producing pipe dream. ■

BACKSEAT DRIVING

It's a warm summer night. Perfect for a drive in the country with some friends. You're in the backseat. Suddenly you're traveling at a high rate of speed, probably faster than you should be going. The sense of being out of control might cause you to laugh. It's a nervous laugh, but it only begins to relieve your tension. Or you might react by tightening every muscle, physiologically attempting to regain control of a situation out of your control. Regardless of your response, you're out of control. Driving somewhere you don't want to go, at a speed faster than you feel comfortable going, is not a pleasant experience.

This is not unlike many practices. Who's in control at your office?

There are many possibilities or combinations: 1) No one's in control; 2) The patients are in control; 3) The staff is in control; 4) Insurance companies are in control; Or 5) The doctor is in control. Which is it?

Control is what we think will finally create calm and fulfillment in our lives. Yet, full control is never possible because we are always a servant to someone or something else. Because of this inescapable fact, we must find a way to obtain joy from the process of serving others while maintaining a healthy balance somewhere between absolute control and total chaos.

Through gritted teeth

Control is to direct and regulate the care a patient receives in the office. In a business setting like this, control does not mean to dominate or coerce. There's the temptation to succumb to this level; it's taught by many management firms who continue to perpetuate a style that worked 10 or 20 years ago and was based on the "do as I say" approach. This dictatorial approach, which often relies on fear tactics, has lost its effectiveness except among the poorly educated and least loyal group of patients. Keeping patients (or staff members) in an agitated state of fear is resented, and while you may seem to get compliance, it comes through gritted teeth.

Without an alternative to the authoritarian style that many doctors find distasteful, all too many doctors are in the back seat of their practices. Besides the frustration and ineffectiveness of being a back seat driver, it causes too many doctors to look for ways to make their million dollars and get out of the profession. If chiropractic is to be the primary mainstream healing art, we need every effective chiropractic doctor committed to a lifetime of service. For some, this will mean rethinking the way the office works to make it a place where you and your staff would be interested in making a career. Interestingly, this revision will make your office a win/win proposition for you and your patients, maybe for the first time!

Depending upon your current state of affairs, you need an action plan to effect this transformation process. Here are some ideas:

1. No one in control. This is a leadership problem. This situation can be recognized by an emergency lifestyle, high staff turnover, low patient retention, and signs of burnout. The doctor has abdicated his or her primary responsibility of leading and directing patients and staff. Clearly, leadership and management skills are a blind spot for most doctors; it's borne out of a low self-image and the short-term strategy best described by a "being-all-things-to-all-people-I-hope-I-don't-offend-anyone" attitude. You must lose the fear that someone might not "like" you.

Action steps. Like many management challenges, this is a self-esteem question. Recognize that no one is going to "build" your practice except you. Recognize that everyone is hoping you'll take a stand and provide direction. Accept the responsibility of having and voicing your opinion! Sit down and list your beliefs; what do you stand for? What personal and chiropractic values will you not compromise under any circumstances? End the chameleon complex that sabotages self respect! Then live by your list with passion.

2. Patients in control. My consulting work in offices and meeting doctors at seminars indicates this is a frequent problem. And guess what? Patients *are* in control and will always be in control! And that's OK. The challenge is to create relationships in which the exchange of chiropractic services is fair and equitable. Until it is, frustration leads to resentment, which leads to anger, which again leads to burnout.

Action steps. Consider changing your office hours so you don't have to be open at both ends of the day, every day. Make sure your staff knows what constitutes an "emergency" so patients aren't taking advantage of your willingness to drop everything on their behalf. If you want to discourage the habit, have the courage to turn away walk-ins, even if you have an opening. Knowingly or unknowingly, you teach patients how to treat you and your office. It starts with the first visit. You are in control of this and other procedural considerations. Yes, there is a price attached to taking control of these issues, but it is surprisingly small if changes are phased in over a period of time and the entire staff is behind their implementation.

3. The staff in control. How many times have I heard a doctor say, "All I want to do is adjust!" Since most chiropractic colleges seem reluctant to teach even fundamental management skills, others have stepped in to fill the vacuum. Most of these are the "I-had-a-huge-prac-tice-you-can-too" schools of management. This outdated approach presupposes similar personalities, values, and long term objectives–an identical match that is rare in a profession made up of "Lone Rangers." Often the doctor abdicates his or her responsibility to an office manager, and "management" becomes merely a spotty enforcement of a written or unwritten staff policy manual. Office management becomes a "black box." Filing a patient's insurance form is a total mystery. Staff accountability is impossible if the doctor doesn't fully understand all aspects of every job function.

Action steps. Get a procedural manual created or updated! Systematize your office procedures in the manual, explaining the what and the how and the *why* of every job function. Make sure every staff member understands and agrees with the long-term objectives of the office. Team members work for the common good of the team. Self-gain power trips, tantrums, or feet dragging should not be permitted by the staff–or the doctor. And if your office uses a computer, the doctor must not be held hostage by a staff member who refuses to cross-train others. Even the doctor should be able to sign on and process records in an emergency. What if your computer person got run over by a bus during the lunch hour?

4. Insurance companies in control. Many veteran doctors are quick to point out that there were many hugely successful practices before chiropractic was recognized by the insurance industry. There are financial, philosophical, and communication challenges that arise by fighting the natural tendency to openly embrace the sickness care outlook extolled by the insurance industry. Financial because, frankly it's easier to make money if you play by their rules. Philosophical, because when you simply treat the patient's symptomatic picture, you are actually practicing medicine, not chiropractic. And communication, because to combat this powerful force requires effective patient communications.

Action steps. Start weaning yourself off insurance cases. Pretty soon, insurance coverage that was seen in the 1980s is going to be gone anyway. When deductibles are regularly $500 or higher or HMOs take over, many offices are going to fail, especially newer doctors who emerged from school with large loans that were secured years ago in a different insurance climate. Create some flexible payment plans or case fee arrangements that can make Initial Intensive Care affordable. Start imagining the day when you won't be accepting insurance or have the overhead associated with it. Actually, it will be a pretty exciting time for chiropractic.

5. Doctor in control. This is what everyone wants. It requires vision, leadership, and courage. And it means being unpopular at times and making optimum care recommendations that can't always be afforded or followed in the real world. The world is hungry for leadership. Effective leadership tends to pull patients and staff to a loftier goal, a higher purpose, and a demand for stricter standards. It helps bring out everyone's best. It puts you in the front seat were you can read the road signs, move confidently through traffic, and take charge.

Action steps. Read some books, especially *The E-Myth, Why Most Businesses Don't Work and What to Do About It* by Michael Gerber. Get some neutral management advice from the many excellent resources of the American Management Association (American Management Association, 135 West 50th Street. New York, NY 10020). Get a management coach. Have lunch with a patient who is in a managerial position or successful small businessperson and pick his or her brain. Develop a "board of directors" to provide ideas, guidance, and direction. Be willing to make mistakes.

Get out of the back seat! Just remember that sharing the chiropractic truth with the world is a process, not a destination. You'll never "get there." However, you will need a map and plenty of energy; why not pack a lunch? ■

THE MYTH OF
PATIENT MANAGEMENT

Perhaps one of the most destructive notions being advanced in chiropractic is that patients can somehow be "managed" into submitting themselves for care.

This is a perspective held by doctors who either distrust patients to respond appropriately or resent the obvious control patients have in the achievement of a doctor's personal and professional goals. So profound is this feeling of lack of control, management specialists have willingly supplied scripted procedures and canned routines to fill the need for everything from cornering patients for the names of friends to "Rambo" recall scripts.

Not only do the questionable techniques that precipitate from the wishful thinking of patient management go against basic tenets of human nature, patients ultimately feel tricked or manipulated, and leave the practice with a bad taste in their mouths. Imagine if these approaches were used by Baskin-Robbins, your car mechanic, or barber!

Does this bad taste contribute to negative word-of-mouth advertising? Does it precipitate the need for models that describe the practice as a "bucket with holes?" Does this cause an insatiable desire for new patients and even more gimmicks to attract them?

What a tangled web we weave...

Attempting to control patients is very stressful. So stressful, in fact, that staff members are hired to perform the strong-arm, high pressure recall techniques. The staff hates it. And so do patients. If it weren't for the fact that it often sabotages the potential for a long-term relationship, it would be a great concept. In fact, when you make patients angry by badgering them for one or two more visits, asking them to divulge a friend's name for a referral, or scolding them for missing an appointment, the effect of negative word-of-mouth can be staggering.

When you buy a lemon

In 1985, Ford Motor Company did a study of their automobile purchasers to discover the impact of negative word of mouth. The study revealed that customers who were happy with their purchases usually told about seven friends. But if someone had bought a lemon, was unhappy with the dealership, or simply upset with the outcome, 22 people heard about it! (Coca-Cola discovered that disgruntled soft drink buyers told twice as many people about their dissatisfaction as did those who were happy when "New Coke" was introduced.)

Negative word of mouth is an effective practice de-builder and it tarnishes the reputation of the entire profession.

Do these manipulative, negative procedures create the voracious appetite for new patients seen in so many offices today? Many offices end up pandering to the least discriminating types of patients, giving away their services, and constantly advertising because their current patients are unwilling to refer others.

Unfortunately, many doctors seem more interested in these short-term solutions. If a new idea or office improvement doesn't pay off in a week or two, there's a desperate sense of nervousness followed by abandonment and search for a new gimmick. Where is the vision? Where is the excitement? Where is the future of chiropractic?

Myopia

Old school chiropractic, with the "aspirin adjustment" perspective, creates a turnstile need for new patients. Combine this with the false assumption that no one wants chiropractic or that a doctor's self-worth is tied to the bottom line or patient volume, and you have a profession looking no further than short-term practice solutions. This myopic vision sabotages credibility, quality, and the excellence needed to increase the impact of chiropractic on humanity and preserve it for future generations of doctors of chiropractic. And their patients.

Manipulative patient management is a short-term perspective. And in "Short-Term Land," the doctor is unsure wellness care is ethical, even though most doctors themselves receive some type of ongoing maintenance care. Is treatment beyond symptomatic relief over-utilization? Is it worth fighting the insurance company who seems to dictate the length of care? Since no one seems to want preventive care, it's seldom offered–especially since it requires communication skills to motivate patients to continue care by paying from their own pocketbooks. Because few patients who come for spinal "repair" work ever understand chiropractic's strong suit–prevention–a self-fulfilling prophecy is created.

Educated patients make better decisions

Enter patient management. With the objective of "improving" patient compliance, fear tactics, manipulative techniques, harassing recall programs, and other procedures are implemented to coerce patients into keeping their appointments or continuing care beyond their own sense of need. It's not surprising that without patient education, patients see these procedures as being financially motivated and only benefiting the doctor. After all, "I'm feeling better now."

Hold onto your wallet!

Whether motivated by financial gain, a statistical goal, real clinical concern, or simply an honest attempt to deliver services the patient should have, the resentment degrades the patient's esteem for the doctor. Whether you're buying a new car, life insurance, or chiropractic care, we all become very suspicious and hold onto our wallets when someone else "has our best interests in mind."

How can you ethically motivate patients to follow through without becoming a high-pressure salesperson? Effective patient education plays a critical role. If patients fully understand the cause, severity, and prognosis of their conditions, then they are no longer dependent upon outside pressure to force them to do what's best. They still may not do what's best, but at least you shed the millstone of monitoring patient compliance because patients have been denied complete information about their conditions.

Isn't the basic issue motivation? Motivation is the technique of tapping into something that is already there. For example, if you go to a seminar and you return home "motivated," you've heard something that struck a responsive chord in you. It was already there. Maybe it caused you to get in touch with some dormant aspect of your value system. Or you heard an affirmation of something you've always believed. The point is, you already had "it" in you and "it" was merely brought to your attention so you could act on it.

Staff motivation works in a similar fashion. If you have a motivated staff, you've created opportunities for them to pursue their personal goals. When you meet a "self-motivated" staff member, you recognize that there's something that makes alignment with practice objectives easy. They already have "it."

Why patients fail

The same is true with patient motivation. Virtually everyone in our culture has been exposed to a health attitude that recognizes that if you have some kind of symptom, you're sick. And when the symptom goes away, you're well. This is an attitude that not only plagues chiropractic, but the medical community as well. Studies at the University of Michigan indicated that as many as 50% to 80% of patients do not follow, or complete, a treatment regimen.

Why?

Howard Leventhal, in his article "Wrongheaded Ideas About Illness" published in the January 1982 issue of *Psychology Today*, suggests several reasons why patients do not comply:

1. To avoid confronting the doctor with their own theories about their condition.

2. To avoid feeling awkward or foolish.

3. To avoid the stress of challenging the doctor.

Medical doctors see these problems when medication isn't taken according to the prescription. You see it in missed appointments. Or patients dropping out the moment they're feeling better. And everyone in the health care community sees it in patients who will not change their lifestyles to prevent their conditions from worsening.

If patient motivation comes from within and compliance is the result of the attitudes, myths, and limited information possessed by the patient, education takes on a new perspective. Patient education can improve patients' understanding of the their problems. Patient education can offer information that can begin the process of changing a patients' health attitudes. Patient education enhances the office's objectives by encouraging an alignment of purpose between the staff and patients. Patient education sets realistic expectations for patients.

Patient education puts the responsibility for patient compliance squarely on the shoulders of the patient. Where it's always been. And always will be. ■

The patient-controlled office

The patient-controlled office is led by a patient-controlled doctor. This well-intentioned doctor takes personal responsibility for each patient "getting it" and following through with what is best for the patient. It's this deep concern and caring attitude that sets the doctor up to be patient controlled. Buying into the patient's problem is a real temptation by professional caregivers. Not that you should coldly offer clinical advice without regard to patients' feelings, but when you assume responsibility with a more than objective professional interest in their conditions, you let patients off the hook, teaching them that their problems are your problems. (If you see their compliance as only a meal ticket or statistic, it *is* your problem!) This "den mother" status sets in motion a whole series of patient management procedures which teach patients that they don't have to take responsibility for themselves. In a sense, this institutionalizes their health, placing unnecessary burdens on the doctor and staff. Strange as it seems, passing up the temptation to be the patient's "friend" can be one of the first steps in shedding the heavy yoke of patient control.

When patients overhear the C.A. making recalls, they learn that some patients don't show up for their appointments, undermining their confidence in the wisdom of keeping their appointments.

The patient-controlled office teaches patients that the doctor's time is not valuable because it too easily accommodates walk-ins.

The patient-controlled office adopts a policy of being available to patients for a grueling 12 or 14 hours a day.

The patient-controlled office has inadvertently communicated to patients that they are buying the doctor's time—not the doctor's talent. Patients expect 14 minutes of the doctor's time and when they don't get it, they get angry or feel shortchanged.

The patient-driven practice

The patient-driven office is significantly different. The doctor and staff recognize they cannot "serve humanity." They have accepted the fact that they won't even meet "humanity." They've chosen a more reasonable approach by focusing their attention on a narrower segment of their community. It sounds impossible from within the grasp of Start Up, but the practice actually grows in size by not trying to be all things to all people. These offices get to know a group of patients which may be distinguished by age, complaint, income, profession, health attitude, or some other qualifier. They enjoy serving this group because of similarities in values, tastes, outlooks on life, or some other common denominator. They learn patients' buying habits, likes and dislikes, where they live, what hours of the day they are available for care, and other aspects of this target market. In this way, patients "drive" the practice in a positive environment based on mutual respect.

Sensitive to the characteristics of this intended market, the doctor outlines the kind of practice he or she wants. The doctor takes an active role in shaping the direction of the practice, by not automatically embracing the status quo simply because, "We've always done it that way before" or "So-and-so up the street doesn't do it this way."

For example, look at the practice hours issue. Not that we should model chiropractic after medicine, but what other health care professional sanctions the exhausting practice hours seen in chiropractic? It may look good on paper, doubling your potential volume by tapping the "rush hours" at both ends of the day, but consider the cost. Typically two overlapping staff positions are needed to cover the entire day. Some staff members don't even know every patient's name! But consider the personal toll on your family relationships and your own life. No wonder so many doctors and staff are experiencing some form of burnout—there's no time for families, hobbies, or a life outside the office.

Get a life!

Here's how one doctor escaped the hours trap. Because he especially enjoyed spending the mornings working out and being with his new family, he wanted to begin practice around 10 a.m. and finish around 7 p.m. in the evening. Going against the textbook formula, as new patients entered the practice, he had their appointments scheduled in the late morning, afternoon, and early evening appointment slots. The few patients that asked for early morning appointments were denied. Gulp.

But there were fewer than he expected. Most new patients have no idea what hours chiropractic doctors keep or should keep. After about three months the roll-over was complete. One day each week he kept the grueling 14-hour schedule to accommodate maintenance patients who had been with him for a long time.

Did he lose any patients? A few. But the satisfaction of having his mornings available for replenishing his energy and having a personal life has been more than worth the cost. Moreover, his practice is growing because he enjoys it for the first time in years and his infectious energy has inspired patients and staff alike.

Hold a patient focus group

One of the techniques used to ferret out the likes and dislikes of your target market is to hold a focus group. Adapted from market research techniques used in the business community, a focus group is an independently supervised meeting of patients. Prior to the session, a list of questions is developed to help reveal information the doctor and staff would like to know. The focus groups I've led have been held during the lunch hour, without anyone from the office in attendance. Six or seven patients, who represent the kinds of patients the doctor is especially interested in serving, are invited to a restaurant or neutral, non-practice location. With their anonymity protected, I stimulate patients to think of their office experience in a new way through a series of rhetorical questions. After about a half hour, when their defenses are down, most patients respond quite openly about various aspects of their office experience. This kind of information is very valuable for making course corrections in office procedure, and usually affirms 80% of what is currently going on.

A focus group session can be led by a trusted patient, business associate, or a close doctor friend from a nearby community. One doctor in Maine decided to get everything out into the open and selected about a dozen ideal patients for a light lunch at the practice and hosted the session himself. He explained that everyone in the room had something in common. As an office they wanted to attract more people like the participants. The reaction was overwhelmingly positive with lots of good ideas being presented. A secondary gain was experienced, too. In the next few weeks, these same patients were responsible for a huge increase in referrals. Participants in a focus group feel a new sense of "ownership" and involvement in the practice. The doctor intends to repeat this process every six or nine months with a new group of patients!

It's important to choose a specific time and setting for patient feedback because, all too often, patients are busy or perceive the doctor is, and they won't volunteer the really good ideas or subtle problems that stand in the way of referrals, or even compliance.

In the patient-driven office, the doctor determines what kinds of services he or she wants to provide that could be perceived as a benefit by the target market and provides them. As the patient-driven office sees more and more patients in alignment with its purpose, it is more willing to refer certain kinds of patients elsewhere. Survival isn't a question anymore. Being held hostage by insurance companies isn't a factor. Having to "sell" chiropractic is no longer necessary.

A common denominator in the stress-free, patient-driven practices I've visited is a systematic patient education program. Education is among the easiest ways to remove the doctor/staff burden of being responsible for patient compliance. It's their health, not yours. When patients actively choose the kind of care they want after fully understanding the nature and severity of the Vertebral Subluxation Complex, the practice becomes a real joy to run. If you neglect to explain fully patients' problems you will have to continue badgering them to keep their appointments.

Running the patient-driven practice is like driving a car. With a destination in mind, you start slowly, pulling into traffic. As you shift gears, your clinical skills respond confidently for you. Entering the passing lane you purr along the countryside, sharing the view and enjoying the journey with others who have discovered this wonderful profession called chiropractic. ■

WHEN DO PATIENTS KNOW ENOUGH?

For many patients, chiropractic is something that happens to them. They are bystanders. They submit to care as long as they experience a sense of progress, the treatment is pleasant, and their insurance company picks up the tab.

They are having their body "serviced" and are often about as involved as when they get a haircut or an oil change.

Other patients are more active participants. They ask intelligent questions. They are aware of their bodies and have integrated their newfound knowledge about chiropractic and health into their lifestyles. It's not that they can hardly wait for their next appointment, but they are pleasant patients to work with and can be prime referral candidates.

High self-esteem

There are other distinguishing characteristics that separate these two groups. Perhaps among the most profound is the patient's level of self worth. Does a patient's self-esteem affect the level of utilization of chiropractic? Most likely it does. Strategies to enhance a patient's self-esteem in your practice would likely improve a patient's chiropractic participation. Yet, like health attitudes, lifestyle, or diet, a patient's self-esteem is the cumulative effect of years of programming.

Besides active listening and other interpersonal skills that communicate your interest in the patient's well being, an aggressive patient education program can have a positive impact on the patient's self-awareness. (A survey published in the January-February issue of *American Health* magazine revealed that medical doctors usually give their patients only 18 seconds to describe their problems before interrupting!) Chiropractic education helps patients better understand their individual potential, places an appropriate value on their care, and gives patients the courage to explain and defend chiropractic outside your office.

The utilization of many products and services is a reflection of a customer's understanding. Once you understand the protocol and know what to do with all the forks, you're more likely to be comfortable in a five-star restaurant. Once you understand how a computer works and what it can do for you, you're more likely to use one.

While we're not likely to find a Restaurant 101 class, have you been in a computer store recently? You'll probably see a video presentation, and every machine will be running a program showing its capabilities and the different kinds of software it can run. These same stores practically give away introductory computer literacy classes and provide free tutorial programs that can be taken home and tried. Computer stores recognize that the more customers know about their products, the more likely they are to buy them, use them, and return to purchase software and peripherals.

Empower the buyer

This happens with many types of first-time purchases: our first VCR, our first home, even our first expensive business suit. The more information the salesperson shared with us, the more we felt involved and empowered to make an intelligent purchase decision. Educating the buyer is one of the primary responsibilities of selling high technology and new ideas, or changing a buyer's attitude. Those who buy without a clear understanding of the product, its uses, or how to get the most out of it suffer from what marketing experts call poor "post-sales satisfaction" or "buyer's remorse." This condition inhibits future purchases, causes customers to hold a negative association with the seller, and results in negative word-of-mouth advertising.

Does this happen in chiropractic?

Of course. There is a vast population suffering from misconceptions about chiropractic. And while you don't have the luxury of having the chiropractic perspective vision hammered into the minds of the public as they watch television every night, you *do* control the environment in which patients receive care. The Herculean task of modifying a patient's belief structure while in your environment is a primary responsibility of every office. Because while chiropractic results may change a patient's *opinion*, a chiropractic education can change a patient's *attitude*. It can equip a patient to speak intelligently about chiropractic or cautiously volunteer, "Well, it worked for me." It can mean the difference between a patient actively referring or dropping out at the first relief of symptoms. It can mean the difference between relief care or a patient bringing in his or her family and pursuing long-term spinal rehabilitation.

Consider every known patient management procedure, technique, fee structure, influence of insurance, patient profile, and every other dimension of chiropractic, and it still goes back to communication. How well are you educating patients so they can make appropriate decisions and place the proper value on the care you give?

Acting "doctorly"

A patient's level of formal education can improve your image as a doctor or lower it. As there are more and more college graduates, the high regard previously afforded those in professional services has diminished. In chiropractic, this problem is worsened by the relative quickness and repetitive nature of the treatments, and the misconception that identical care is administered to all patients. "How can something that's done so quickly be so difficult to do or cost so much?" reasons a patient. "That was the most expensive two and a half minutes I've ever experienced," another patient thinks to himself.

Many patients are kept in the dark during the initial examination. Tests are not explained while they are being administered and comments are reduced to a knowing, "Uhmmm," attempting to heighten the dramatic importance of the eventual report of findings. Perhaps this works with some patients, but without an open dialogue, teaching patients and helping them place a value on your expertise, you are overlooking an excellent educational opportunity. Later, patients have a better basis for the doctor's clinical recommendations and the effectiveness of the report of findings is less dependent upon the doctor's ability to present his or her "opinion." Without a clear understanding of how recommendations are reached, patients rely more heavily on their own notions of health. Foreshadow your report of findings by revealing your findings as you conduct your examination.

Similarly, without the proper chiropractic education, patients undervalue post-symptomatic relief care. As patients compare the cost with the relief and sense of progress they experienced during Initial Intensive Care, they are inclined to equate a lower value with Reconstructive Care because the results are not as dramatic. Without a targeted communication plan, this discrepancy in perceived value (cost/benefit) forces a patient to re-evaluate the need for continued care. This problem is compounded because it often occurs simultaneously with discontinued insurance coverage. Patient education, when combined with a thoughtful wellness fee structure, can help combat this perceived decrease of return on investment.

Aside from the immediate benefits of a well-informed patient base, fewer inappropriate questions, and patients who follow through because they understand a bigger vision of chiropractic, effective patient education creates a legacy. Educated patients are patients who can explain chiropractic well enough and accurately enough to inspire their friends and families.

Patient education is the key

Merely experiencing results is not enough. What about the hundreds of thousands of patients who have gotten results—but have never mentioned chiropractic to their friends? Perhaps their reluctance is based on a lack of information or the inability to persuasively articulate how and why chiropractic works—again, the result of ineffective patient education. Educated patients can be more effective chiropractic ambassadors in your community than expensive television commercials, free services, or other non-therapeutic marketing incentives. Educated patients can personalize their approach to prospective referrals. Educated patients can answer questions. Educated patients have information that gives them a base of power and confidence–not only to continue their care beyond insurance coverage, but to share their knowledge with others.

Even the very first doctors recognized the educational aspects of their profession. After all, the word doctor comes from the Latin, *docere*, meaning "to teach" or "to cause to accept." Perhaps this has even more significance today in the Information Age. To practice without using every educational tool, technique, or technology to educate patients is to hinder their understanding of their condition and the motivation necessary to take responsible action.

When do patients know enough? When they enroll in chiropractic college, of course. ■

A REPORT ON THE
REPORT OF FINDINGS

Members of the baby boom generation are increasingly showing up in chiropractic offices these days. This is the generation that drove Volkswagens in 60's and 70's with bumper stickers that said, "Question Authority." They're seeking second opinions. They're asking more questions than the generation before them. Their questions are similar to the questions asked by their four year old offspring: Why?

While it is beneficial in building patient rapport to explain what the examinations reveal as you're conducting them, answering most patient questions are reserved for the report of findings.

Amazingly, some doctors do not consistently give a report of findings. Left in the dark, patients must rely solely on how they feel as a guideline for their length of care. Rather than practicing chiropractic, the office assumes a medical posture as patients come and go, seeking drug-free, non-surgical relief of pain. This reduces the patient's benefit from chiropractic care by sabotaging an understanding of its preventive and wellness role in optimum health.

For doctors who recognize the benefits of improved compliance and follow through by educating their patients, the report of findings becomes the cornerstone in their systematized approach. Here are some techniques today's best communicators are using to maximize the full impact of their report of findings:

1. Use pictures. We are visual animals. We get most of our information about the world around us through our eyes. We remember images much longer than words. Virtually all of us are carrying around perfect images of Neil Armstrong stepping onto the surface of the moon. Images last. For patients, especially those raised on television, making your report more visual can have a significant impact on patient understanding. X-rays, spinal models, and wall posters are often used. But have you considered using pictures that illustrate the five components of the Vertebral Subluxation Complex? To help patients understand the spinal kinesiopathology you could use pictures of someone wearing braces (loss of normal motion or position), the tin man from the Wizard of Oz (stiff and not moving properly), the leaning tower of Piza, or a picture of a worn tire caused by the front end of a car out of alignment. Using metaphors and visualizations of key concepts can help patients from a wide variety of socio-economic and educational backgrounds understand this new approach to health called chiropractic.

2. Use a consistent structure. Unlike Olympic diving judges, patients don't hold up score cards at the end of your report. You can't be sure how well you connected with your patient during the report for months later. By then it's difficult to remember what you said and what order you said it in. Adopt some type of consistent structure, starting with a review of the symptoms that prompted the patient's investigation of chiropractic and ending with a call to action. Use this skeleton outline of topics and personalize it for each patient by revealing your examination findings and treatment approach. This will keep you on track and avoid some of the time-consuming tangents and meanderings that often occur when you sense the patient isn't "getting it."

3. Avoid the X-ray view box monologue. The temptation is to turn a majority of the report into a stand up routine in front of the X-ray view box. Patients are intrigued by this view of their bodies and it is easy to squander valuable time explaining the heart shadow, intestinal gas bubbles, and the meaning of all the lines and angles you've drawn. Worse, the static views taken in most offices tend to reinforce the notion that the patient's problem is merely a bone out of place. Since flexion/extension and other dynamic views of the spine can be difficult for patients to understand, this simplistic "bone out of alignment" notion can lead patients to think just a few adjustments will be necessary. Spend as little time as possible at the X-ray view box and concentrate on an explanation of the muscles and soft tissues involved that justify the necessity of non-symptomatic rehabilitative and wellness care.

4. Answer the four questions. Patients begin your report of findings with four basic questions, What's wrong with me? Can chiropractic help? If so, how long will it take? How much will it cost? You can put patients at ease and anticipate their unspoken concerns by telling them at the beginning that "most of our patients come to our office with four basic questions..." and explain that you will "...answer these four questions along with any other questions you may have..."

When answering the first question, you're correlating the symptomatic picture the patient can relate to with your examination findings. As you answer the second question, you're explaining what chiropractic care will involve in their case, such as the adjusting approach, any adjunctive procedures, visit frequency, etc. As you answer the third question you must give some type of reasonable expectations as to how long before the patient will know that their decision to select your office was a good one. How long before some type of relief can be expected? How long for the completion of rehabilitation? What can the patient do to participate and speed their own recovery? The fourth question is usually avoided by doctors, however, my experience suggests that offices with excellent compliance and high patient visit averages are offices in which the doctor addresses finances.

5. Explain how long the report will be. This is an often overlooked piece of information that, when volunteered, can serve to improve rapport and participation. How long should a report be? My experience in successful chiropractic offices suggests that if your report is non-existent or less than 10 minutes, you're probably not giving the patient enough information to fully appreciate the nature and severity of their problem. Longer than 20 minutes and you're numbing the patients with too much detail.

6. Offer facts. If you want to avoid "selling" chiropractic care, you must offer facts and let the patient decide what they want. This is no place for scare tactics, yet you have an obligation to explain the severity of their spinal degeneration or the likely affects of neglecting their problem. The key is to offer facts that make sense to the patient and allows them to stay in control of their health. Selling patients something they don't want or understand results in buyer's remorse and ultimately damages your clinical credibility and word-of-mouth advertising about your office.

7. Involve the patient. While this is your time to shine and the spotlight is on you, ask questions along the way to test their assimilation of the material. The most obvious opportunity for involvement is to have the patient identify which phase of Subluxation Degeneration their spine is in at the X-ray view box. "I'd like you to compare your neutral lateral cervical view with one of these examples here. Which phase comes closest to matching yours?" Motivation comes from involvement. If you want motivated patients you must seek ways to get them involved in their case so your report doesn't become a lecture.

8. Give optimum treatment plan. By the time of the report, most doctors have an idea about the patient's financial resources or transportation problems that could interfere with their care. Taking these suspicions into consideration, many doctors present a less-than-optimum treatment plan to increase the chances of it being accepted on its first presentation. Not only is this not fair to the patient, it's presumptuous. How do you know that they don't value their health enough to get a loan? Or would be willingly make special provisions to get to your office at the visit frequency you recommend? Present your optimum recommendations, then negotiate modifications if necessary.

9. Outline patient responsibilities. Patients won't regain their health with simply your single-handed efforts alone! They must keep their appointments. They need to report reinjuries. They probably need to make modifications to their lifestyles. What other responsibilities do you want patients to assume? Give cancellation notice? Refer others? Attend an orientation class? This is the time to outline them.

10. Present a tool to help them explain to others. There are countless people your patient will encounter who haven't seen the X-rays or heard your report. You must empower your patients to explain and defend their chiropractic decision to others outside your sphere of influence. Of course, the spouse or parent should be at the report. If they can't, equip your patients with a document or report they can take home to replicate your explanation to others. If you don't, many patients will be talked out of care. It should not contain the technical stuff that moves insurance companies! Remove the jargon. Instead of "cervical range of motion examination results" how about something like "you were unable to rotate your head to the left by about 15 degrees less than you were able to rotate it to the right."

These ten points can help you present a more powerful report of findings. Yet the first step to take is to begin tape recording your reports and listening to them. It's excruciating to listen to yourself speak, however it's an easy way to enhance your single most important patient communication. ■

MENTORING PATIENTS TO HEALTH

A famous psychologist was asked how he got his patients to change and emerge from their psychological problems—why some patients eventually seem to get well and others didn't change. Was it, the interviewer queried, the result of the patients finally understanding their problems well enough to transcend beyond them? "No," he said, "if that were true, all any one of us would have to do is read books and we would assume the wisdom of the ages." Look at the countless how-to-lose-weight books. Most overweight people own plenty.

Then how do patients change? "Through relationships," he observed. "As doctors, we mentor patients to wellness through our relationships with them." The quality of that healing relationship affects compliance, speed of recovery, and ultimately the referral process.

Isn't it interesting that the patients you especially enjoy serving seem to get well sooner? What does it take to build a relationship that can serve as an effective vehicle to mentor someone through symptomatic relief and into a preventive chiropractic lifestyle? Here are some points to consider when you begin a relationship with your next new patient:

Share common goals. While more and more of today's chiropractic patients have lost confidence in medical solutions to their problems, chiropractic still hasn't shed its "bad back doctor" image. The goal of some chiropractic doctors is simply to improve the symptomatic picture. Others see each new patient as an opportunity to create a lifetime relationship–from symptomatic relief through rehabilitation and into some type of ongoing maintenance relationship. Symptomatic relief relationships are the easiest because it is the relationship most new patients have in mind when they begin care. When doctors take the path of least resistance, they place themselves on a new patient treadmill, always looking for more new patients while overlooking the clinical necessity and patient benefits of preventive chiropractic care.

Doctors with a longer vision in mind recognize that they must acknowledge the patient's limited vision during the initial phases of care. These doctors recognize that they must "earn the right" to discuss maintenance care by first relieving the patient's symptomatic picture. You must give patients what they *want* before you can ever have the chance to give them what they *need*. The value of rehabilitative and maintenance care can be shared on subsequent visits.

This is when a patient's familiarity with the five components of the Vertebral Subluxation Complex is so helpful. When patients understand that their problem is more serious than a bone out of place and are aware that muscle and soft tissue damage and calcium salt deposition can be present without symptoms, it brings understanding to the old adage, "Once you start chiropractic you have to go for the rest of your life."

When in doubt, ask

If the doctor and patient share similar goals because of mutual understanding, there is an increased likelihood that the easy goal of symptomatic relief will be achieved and higher health goals can be set. One way to find out what outcomes your new patients want is to ask.

What results do they want? A temporary patch job? Prevention? Optimum health? How much energy are they willing to give the relationship? Keeping appointments, doing exercises, changing their lifestyle, etc. How long will they suspend judgment and follow through before they expect results? One visit? Five visits? Ten visits? Create a relationship in which your new patients feel comfortable in honestly revealing their expectations. Reduce patient drop-out and increase the chance of making a difference by sharing common goals. Get it out into the open. Make both parties accountable.

Share a common language. This is related to goal setting, yet recognizes the difference between the chiropractic doctor's expertise and the new patient's beginner status. Whether it's the relationship between a computer expert and a computer rookie or between a car mechanic and its driver, this difference can cause problems. It's difficult to build a meaningful relationship with someone from a foreign country who has different customs and speaks a different language. It's the same with patients who show up in your office. They speak a dialect heavily influenced by aspirin commercials, knee-jerk tonsillectomies, and bottles of pink antibiotics.

The understanding of bodily functions and the language to describe them are almost non-existent among even the best educated. Yet, many of your "ideal" patients, with whom you can most quickly build a relationship, are very aware of their bodies and well-being. You must supply the language skills to help patients fully appreciate the nature and severity of their conditions. Certainly this is one of the real values of having a systematized patient education program in your office. Not only does it give patients a chiropractic model for understanding the true nature of health, it should also supply the language needed to describe their health complaint to you, and what chiropractic is to others. Otherwise, chiropractic is simply something that *happens* to them and a nurturing relationship never evolves.

Patient education makes better patients. Think back to the acute patient with whom you aborted your normal educational routines. I'll bet he or she dropped out early. Systematize your efforts so you can impart at least a rudimentary level of chiropractic science and philosophy without expending large amounts of energy. Long-term relationships require that the parties speak similar languages.

Fair exchange. A doctor/patient relationship costs money. There is a business relationship as well as a health mentoring relationship. Ignoring this reality sets a doctor up for disappointment and burnout. To continue this type of relationship there must be a fair exchange between both parties. Patients purchase value from your office. The cost (price, time, inconvenience of repeated visits, etc.) must be less than the benefit received (pain relief, improved self-image, regained abilities, etc.) When this cost/benefit ratio dips below a fair exchange, expect a change in the relationship.

A good example of this is when patients start feeling better and are cut off from their insurance benefits. Money is a factor. This cruel economic reality is often difficult for doctors who receive their care without any impact to their monthly budget to appreciate. Ever wonder why every patient you've ever treated isn't still showing up once or twice a month for a wellness visit? If it's a choice between a pizza and movie with the kids or an adjustment when they're feeling fine, guess which one they choose?

Offices that boast patient visit averages in the 50s, 60s and higher have some type of wellness fee structure in place to accommodate this change in perceived value. An affordable fee structure won't completely avoid patient drop-out; however, it improves the opportunity to continue a healing relationship into rehabilitative and maintenance stages of care.

Set a good example. It sounds so obvious, but is it? It's the 1990s and there is still a sizable contingent of doctors and staff members who smoke! Even worse, there are doctors and staff members who are not under regular chiropractic care themselves. It's the health care equivalent of the cobbler's children going without shoes. Overweight? Lose it. Shabby office? Remodel it. Facial hair? Trim it. Bad breath? Fix it. Patients are incredibly sensitive to the health habits of their doctor. To mentor someone to health, you need to be healthy yourself.

Thousands of patients who could be helped never make it into your office because they don't recognize the role of the nervous system and its relationship to the spine and overall health. And while it's difficult to reach those not in your office, it is the responsibility of every doctor and staff member to use the mentoring process to change the perception and understanding of every patient who *does* make it into your office. Only then is there any hope for a meaningful, long-term relationship. ■

GROWING
CHIROPRACTIC CLIENTS

While many chiropractic doctors continue to toil under the sickness model of health care, taking the path of least resistance by looking to insurance companies to dictate the length of care, more and more offices are taking a different path. As more doctors recognize the wellness and preventive nature of chiropractic, they are stabilizing their practices, reducing stress, and getting off the new patient treadmill by *keeping* more of the patients that they do get.

In chiropractic circles, it is well accepted that some type of ongoing chiropractic care is beneficial. Even if not familiar with the clinical research suggesting maintenance care, most doctors and their staffs receive some type of ongoing care. When chiropractic care is readily available and schedules permit, most chiropractic doctors get adjusted about once a week. Even doctors who look to insurance companies for case management guidance receive regular non-symptomatic adjustments. Sometimes our schedules are too hectic, or the willing hands of an associate or reciprocating doctor aren't readily available. Yet, your patients would probably benefit from some type of ongoing chiropractic care in the same way you do.

The new patient solution

What if 30% or more of all the patients you've ever seen over the years came in for a wellness visit on the same visit frequency you enjoy?

You would no longer have a voracious appetite for new patients. In fact, you'd be scouring the colleges for associate doctors to help handle the demand! Suddenly, you'd have a stable, predictable practice that would enable you to take vacations and have a life outside your office. Your non-symptomatic "well" patients could easily schedule their visits around your week-long vacations and frequent three-day family outings. Your practice would still be intact when you returned.

Going back to the Latin root of the word patient, *patior,* meaning "to suffer," these wellness-oriented individuals wouldn't be patients in the traditional sense. They certainly wouldn't be suffering! Quite the opposite. People (like you) who receive some type of ongoing non-symptomatic chiropractic care are active, vital, and make a difference in the lives of countless others they influence. Rather than patients, maybe you would think of them as chiropractic "clients."

The doctor/client relationship is different than the doctor/patient relationship. Patients have a short-term outlook (get me out of pain). Clients enjoy a long-term perspective. Patients look at chiropractic care as something that happens to them. Clients are in touch with their bodies and want to optimize their health. Patients see health as a destination. Clients see health as a process. While the miracle cures and easily documentable progress of Initial Intensive Care are fulfilling in a super-ficial sense, chiropractic patients aren't as much fun to be around as clients. The client relationship is more of a partnership approach to health, with open lines of communication. The adversarial "prove it works" attitude is gone. In fact, when a patient becomes a client, the visit-to-visit dialogue becomes less and less health oriented!

Chiropractic clients are grown from chiropractic patients. Not every patient is available to become a client, but that doesn't stop offices with this vision from taking active measures to introduce and encourage preventive, chiropractic lifestyles on the part of every new patient. Here are a few of the ingredients found in successful offices:

Chiropractic science. A common denominator of every office with a sizable wellness practice is an acquaintance with research substantiating the necessity of continued joint mobilization for the prevention of spinal degeneration and supporting muscle scar tissue.

Chiropractic philosophy. An underpinning of these doctors' scientific background is a well-grounded chiropractic philosophy. While they don't beat their patients over the head with their beliefs or scold patients for an occasional use of aspirin, their philosophy is evident in the answers given to everyday patient questions. This philosophy helps doctors combat the continual influence of the medical "sickness" model of health from patients, insurance companies, and drug advertising on television.

Patient education. These offices have a systematized way of communicating chiropractic science and philosophy to their patients. They use every opportunity while their patients are within their sphere of influence to enlarge their vision of health. Yes, they use videos, brochures, and educational sign-in sheets, but they also give spinal care classes and have some type of continuing patient dialogue on every visit. They recognize that a single super-duper report of findings can't overcome a lifetime of being indoctrinated by the medical model of health.

Acknowledge patient motives. Doctors with a large number of well patients don't fool themselves. They recognize that most patients do not begin care with the idea of starting a lifelong relationship. And they also recognize that on the first couple of visits they have not earned the right to ask or expect a long-term commitment. The value of long-term care is gently introduced as patients start feeling better.

Feedback loops. Successful well-patient practices have well developed feedback loops to obtain patient perceptions about the practice, procedures, and personalities. They keep in touch with current patients by holding frequent focus groups, using patient questionnaires, and on the 10th or 15th visit take the pulse of patients' attitudes about the office and their care. When patients drop out of care, there is a non-judgmental mechanism to uncover the patients' motives for discontinuing care that can help prevent the problem or situation from occurring with future patients.

Role models. These offices are proud of their high patient retention and communicate this idea of "success" to their patients. Instead of the typical symptomatic "it-worked-for-me" relief testimonials in the reception room, patient testimonials in these offices stress the wellness and preventive aspects of care. You'll find case histories on X-ray view boxes and "Patient of the Month" profiles emphasize why patients have decided to continue with the chiropractic after Relief Care. The notion that chiropractic works is practically taken for granted.

Wellness fees. Virtually every office with large numbers of wellness patients (and especially children) have some type of post-symptomatic, post-insurance financial plan. These offices recognize that most insurance doesn't cover wellness and preventive care, and they are realistic about what a family can afford to pay for their care when they're feeling fine and have exhausted insurance benefits.

Rewarding referrals. Birds of a feather flock together and offices interested in developing their wellness client base know that their patients have friends and relatives who share the same wellness attitudes. They identify these "ideal" patients and make special efforts to nurture and reward their kept appointments and referrals.

Stimulating environment. Since they expect their well patients to return to the office countless times over the months and years of their client relationship, these offices are fun places to be. The office environment is creative and stimulating. Not only are the magazines up to date, but so are the colors, carpet, lighting, and accessories. While not necessarily interior design showcases, they have a homey, yet professional tone that is enticing and always features something new and different. Bulletin boards are changed regularly. The children's toy box receives new additions. And reading material is uplifting, highly visual, and reflects a healthy, optimistic outlook.

These are just a few of the attributes found in offices that get a lot of new patients—and are keeping them in the 1990s. As insurance coverages continue to decline and deductibles rise, keeping patients will become as important as getting them. Just about any chiropractic doctor can achieve symptomatic improvement. One of the ways to measure success in this decade will be how many patients you can grow into chiropractic clients. ■

IDENTIFYING YOUR IDEAL PATIENT

Whether I'm working with chiropractic doctors, CPAs, advertising agencies or other small professional businesses, each has a type of ideal patient, client, or project they particularly enjoy. Typically, these are situations characterized by a win/win environment and a mutual respect between the buyer and seller.

Imagine your entire practice filled with "Ideal Patients."

Rather than aiming for some arbitrary and escalating *quantity* of patients, many offices are now directing their attention to improving the *quality* of their patients. Quality is defined differently by each practice. But how do you change your patient mix to reflect more of the kinds of "quality" patients you would especially enjoy serving? Better question: should you?

You must decide that it's appropriate to actively have a hand in shaping the composition of your patient profile. There are doctors who have interpreted their professional obligation to include serving virtually anyone who can dial seven digits on a telephone and present their spines in the office. Conversely, if you have the capacity to serve those seeking care, and you denied access to chiropractic due to some arbitrary social standard, that would be wrong, too. What many offices are doing is simply identifying characteristics of those patients they especially enjoy serving, and making a specific effort to attract them.

What types of patients do you enjoy serving? What are their common denominators? Is it their health attitudes? Personality? Income? Occupation? Hobbies? Lifestyle? Personal habits? Age? Cash? Insurance? Insurance company? Condition?

What is it about your special patients that makes them special?

In an office I consulted with, the doctor enjoyed working with young professionals, especially those who were active and sports-minded. Conflict mounted as the C.A. paid extra attention to elderly patients, making them feel especially welcome in the office while often neglecting the young professionals, in effect sabotaging the kinds of patients the doctor wanted to see. We each have our own particular social orientation, shaped by our background and personalities, and patients feel most comfortable when the office is in alignment. The C.A.'s actions were the source of constant frustration and the problem had to be permanently resolved. (The C.A. is now happily working in a senior citizen facility.)

The struggle facing staff members was more serious in an accounting firm I consulted with. After three years, the practice had plateaued. During a brainstorming session, it was revealed that one of the two principals wanted to have the largest accounting firm in the state. The other, stunned by this discovery, mumbled something about wanting to have fewer clients with interesting accounting problems that could be served in a smaller, "boutique" setting with a low overhead. With their "hidden agendas" out in the open, they continued to practice together but with separate kinds of clients. Unfortunately, the motives, expectations, and attention required to serve these two different types of clients levied a high toll on the staff, who were placed in the position of "choosing sides." Nine months later, they formally separated. Neither one was right or wrong in their vision of the ideal practice and the kind of client to be served. They just had different visions. Today they are both doing well and experiencing greater success and fulfillment than when they were together.

A common complaint I hear among doctors is having to "sell" chiropractic to patients. Many offices have stopped selling chiropractic.

They have begun to *market* chiropractic. And the difference is more than semantic. Selling focuses on the needs of the seller, marketing on the needs of the buyer. Selling is preoccupied with the seller's need to convert his time and services into cash. Marketing is the idea of identifying and satisfying the needs of the customer. It's the difference between selling 1/4" drill bits versus supplying a solution for those who want to make 1/4" holes. Selling is difficult, marketing is difficult, but for different reasons—primarily motivation.

If you're merely "selling" a drill bit, anyone with $1.69 becomes a qualified buyer. If you're "marketing" drill bits, you need to first identify those who need holes. Particular kinds of holes. In what types of materials. You have to find out what a customer wants. And when a customer asks for a way to make 1" square holes and you don't have a solution you make a referral to another source.

You must identify the kinds of patients for whom you have solutions. The temptation is to say everyone with a spine! But you can't be all things to all people. No matter what you think, you aren't providing the same high level of care to patients who are skeptical, have negative attitudes, or poor personal hygiene. It's human nature to search out those who are appreciative, responsive, and open.

Identify the characteristics of the ideal patient interested in the kind of care you provide, and then focus your efforts on nurturing and expanding the number of these kinds of patients in your practice. You may discover that the unique factors in your ideal patient transcend age, sex, income, occupation, and other typical demographic qualifiers. Maybe your ideal patient fits a particular "attitudinal" description. One doctor who especially enjoyed working with young professionals joked that many of his favorite patients wore Rockport shoes! The cars parked in front of the computer store are generally foreign built. In front of the bowling alley? American. What do your ideal patients have in common?

Begin to shape your practice so it is especially responsive to the needs of the kinds of patients you want. What kind of magazines do they like to read? Do they have children who need to be entertained? Is the waiting room furniture easy for older patients to rise up out of? Do busy professionals quietly resent being handed a clipboard and a bent pen on their first visit? Do certain patients want better explanations about X-ray exposure? When you begin marketing chiropractic instead of selling it, you simply make it easier for the kinds of patients you want to feel comfortable in your practice.

More often than not, your ideal patient shares your value system. In fact, I was recently identified by my dentist as someone who shared the same value system with him and his staff. I received an excellent letter from them. While the letter consisted of only six sentences, it mentioned that the dentist and the staff had recently discussed "the kinds of patients we especially enjoy having in our practice," and that in general, "these patients share similar values with the dental staff." Further, they indicated, "because of this similar value system, people you like are very likely to be the kinds of people we would like, too." And since they would like to build an entire practice of people like me, if the opportunity should ever arise for me to send someone to them, they would be especially grateful. What a wonderful referral tool. No selling. No stress. No arm twisting. It was a compliment to me that they valued my judgment and thought that I would send them the "right" kind of patient. Guess what I'll do next time the subject of dental care comes up in conversation?

Who are your ideal patients? ■

WORTHY
OF CARE

Cliches are dangerous because they over-simplify or generalize the truth in such sweeping ways we forget to question their implications. However, "Birds of a feather flock together" is not one of these deceptive cliches. It rings true. Especially when it comes to referrals.

When I work with doctors to help them create the practice they want, we inevitably talk about the kinds of patients they particularly like serving. I imagine every doctor's dream practice is to have it full of Ideal Patients. For the new practitioner, an Ideal Patient is anyone with a spine who can get it to the office. For others, it's anyone who has a spine and pays their bill. And for others, it's merely a willingness to comply. It often varies depending upon how far the doctor has progressed in his or her own economic survival.

The nightmare patient

Many offices are plagued with what some might call "Nightmare Patients." These are patients who don't respect your time or your talent. These are the patients that we let ruin an otherwise wonderful day. With enough of them in your practice, you can start believing that chiropractic would be a great profession—if it weren't for patients.

Because birds of a feather flock together, when the Nightmare Patient feels compelled to refer friends or family to your office, you discover that the meaning of the word "clone" pre-dates genetic engineering! The corollary to this phenomenon is the headache patient referring the headache patient and the lower back patient referring the lower back patient. If 5% of your current patient base is Nightmare Patients, you're stuck with this patient mix–unless you intervene and take active measures to change it.

Do Nightmare Patients receive the same level of time and attention from you and your staff as your Ideal Patients do? Probably not.

There is a finite number of patients who can be seen in any given day, week, month, year, or career. Why not increase the number of Ideal Patients in your patient mix so you'll have more fun, do a better job, and make more of an impact in your community? But how?

List your ideal patients

First, define your Ideal Patient. Probably the biggest reason most of us are unhappy is because we haven't stopped to determine what we want. At your next staff meeting have everyone write down their own list of Ideal Patients. They don't even necessarily have to be active patients. What you're looking for are real people who personify attributes that make them Ideal. Four or five names will do. Then have everyone share their lists, explaining why they've included each patient. This is a valuable exercise that facilitates communication between the staff and doctor. Discover the qualities each staff member considers important in the profile of an Ideal Patient. It's interesting how it often varies depending on job responsibility. Even more interesting, these patients probably receive an extraordinarily high level of service.

Doing this exercise can help you avoid what happened in an office in which the doctor especially enjoyed working with children. During a staff meeting I facilitated, we brainstormed everyone's ideas of their Ideal Patients. After listing six or seven patient names, they compared notes. During this exercise we discovered the front desk assistant didn't like children! She didn't like the mess they made of the reception room and didn't like being a babysitter. Ultimately she had to move on in her career as the doctor expanded the pediatric side of his practice.

Having brainstormed the attributes of the typical Ideal Patient with doctors and staff at seminars, I've discovered that Ideal Patients range in age from newborns to grandpas. Male, female, white collar, blue collar, rich, poor; there isn't a clear cut demographic describing the Ideal

Patient. But there do seem to be attitudinal characteristics. They are often described as open-minded, aware, health-conscious, coachable, enthusiastic, educated, willing to take responsibility, conscientious, self-confident, and what the Santa Monica, California think tank Rand Corporation describes as being "inner-directed." These are values that transcend community size, geographic location, and nationality.

I believe all these qualities are simply ways of saying Ideal Patients have a high level of self-esteem.

Based on this observation, you have two choices if you're interested in building a practice full of Ideal Patients. The first is to attract patients who already have a high level of self-esteem by using a variety of marketing approaches within and outside the practice.

The other is to "grow" Ideal Patients from among your current patient base by enhancing patients' self-esteem each time they have an office encounter. Just as patients' acute symptoms can disguise their true personalities during the early part of care, the fact that patients are in a doctor's office may distort their self-image. Happily, this is something you can change—a change that may have profound long-term effects beyond an improvement in their physical health.

Self-esteem can be defined as thinking of oneself with respect. Without discipline and compassion, it becomes destructive pride. Our self-esteem is the image we hold of ourselves, affecting our ability to enjoy life and contribute to others. Low self-esteem, often the result of programming by our parents as a child, holds us back for the rest of our lives. "Be careful." "Take it easy." "You can't do that!" "No!" And a million other subtle forms of programming shaped our self-image "tape loops." How we think of ourselves shapes every aspect of our lives, including our lifestyle, personal hygiene, and our worthiness in spending money (on ourselves) with a health care provider.

That's a major point. What's chiropractic worth? And am I worth it? Am I worth it beyond what my insurance policy seems to think is necessary? A high level of self-esteem (and money) is necessary to persevere beyond relief care only.

One way to increase someone's self-esteem is to consult child development books that explain how to develop this valuable trait in children. Then adapt the techniques into practical things you and your staff can do with patients. Here are some practical examples you can start implementing today:

Run on time. A frequent patient complaint is waiting to see the doctor. An office that runs on time, respecting the value of the patients' time, is an absolute must. Your time is valuable–so is a patient's.

Office environment. Investing in contemporary, comfortable office furniture and accessories tells patients you value them. Don't buy into the "they-don't-want-me-to-look-too-successful" myth! Of course, avoid the marble entry way and the chandeliers, but invest in your patients and their office experience. Show them they're worthy of chiropractic care.

Reward referrals. If you've ever seen patients count the names on your sign in sheet and mentally multiply the cost of care, you already know why you need to say thank you with something more than a pre-printed "Thank-You Gram" created in 1967. "Thank you" and "please" are two words you can't say loud enough or often enough.

Praise patients. Anyone entering your office has recognized the value of the care you provide. Avoid scolding anyone for anything. Didn't do your exercises? No problem. Didn't come in last week like you were scheduled? No problem. Praise patients for recognizing the need to see you at all. Identify ways the patient would benefit by complying with your recommendations. "It'll help you regain your health faster," or "It'll help prevent your problem from returning," etc.

If every patient continued to feel better, and feel better about themselves simply by being in your office, your retention statistics would soar. There's plenty of evidence showing the relationship between psychological health and physical health. Ignoring either thwarts complete recovery. Touching a patient's self esteem is a good way to ensure that you'll have the chance to touch his or her spine for rest of their life. ■

AN EFFECTIVE
REFERRAL DIALOGUE

As the most influential medium on earth, word-of-mouth advertising is also the most difficult to create and control. Perhaps that's why it's so potent. Yet word-of-mouth advertising is the primary source of referrals. And, thankfully, it is considerably less expensive to produce and implement than television commercials and other exotic forms of advertising. There are active steps you can take to enhance the kind of referrals you receive and shape the direction of your practice through word-of-mouth advertising. I call this process the referral dialogue.

Hollywood knows better than perhaps any other industry the value of word-of-mouth advertising. With ballooning production budgets, studios cannot afford to actively advertise their latest releases over the weeks and months of a typical first-run showing. Their strategy is to attract only the first weekend's audience. To "prime the pump." Hollywood has learned that no amount of advertising can prop up a poor picture. Word-of-mouth advertising has become an integral part of their marketing efforts.

Similarly, no matter how strong the lure of chiropractic advertising, it cannot overcome significant internal management problems, lack of results, staff negativity, or other crucial aspects of a professional practice. The fact is, effective word-of-mouth advertising is the marketing foundation for most practices.

Just as a movie must be "good" to sustain a continued screening, so too must you get good clinical results. As a basis for the following concepts, let's assume you get excellent results and your office procedures create a warm, friendly environment with a clear purpose.

It is somewhat of an axiom that the quality of a referral is a reflection of who's doing the referring. Skeptical patients refer fellow skeptics. Personal injury cases refer personal injury victims. Deadbeats refer deadbeats. That being true, if you're not happy with aspects of your current patient mix, how do you break this vicious cycle?

Would you like more PI cases or more cash cases? More families and children? Maybe you'd like to work with fewer symptomatic patients. Or maybe you especially enjoy difficult or unusual cases, but can't seem to find them. If members of your current patient mix continue to refer those like themselves, you're trapped. The referral dialogue is one way to begin affecting a change in your practice mix and modifying the kinds of referrals you get.

Can your staff recognize your ideal patient?

There are two practical aspects to this effort. First, you must decide what kind of patients you really want. What are their needs and attitudes? Where do they live? How do they think? What time of the day are they available for care? And on and on. This isn't a 10-minute exercise written on a napkin while you're waiting for your lunch to arrive! If you're sincerely interested in changing the status quo, you must take the time to get "inside" your intended market. While this may be as easy as visualizing a composite picture with the aspects of several of your favorite patients, that's just the beginning. It's crucial that the doctor's vision be shared with the staff so everyone understands the objective and specifics of this new targeted effort. Everyone needs to be able to recognize new "ideal" patients when they call on the phone or walk in the door! Everyone needs to know what kind of patient, what kind of symptoms, and what kind of attitudes are embodied in your ideal patient. It's the only way you can begin filling your practice with the kinds of patients you want.

The second element is the actual articulation of the benefits you offer this market and actively sharing them. You must take the time to write down the words, concepts, and phrases that describe the kind of patient or the kinds of conditions you're hoping to increase in your practice. Share these ideas with the entire staff. Then, when the opportunity presents itself, share these descriptions with patients. Only then will your patients have the words you want used to describe what you do. Then when a referral opportunity presents itself to them, there is a better chance that they will be using your words. Especially if it's different from the kind of care you provided them or the condition for which they originally came for treatment.

Sowing ideal patients

For example, a patient is signing in at the front desk and mentions to the C.A., "I haven't had a headache all week; the doctor has really helped me." The C.A., knowing that one of the doctor's goals is to increase the number of children in the practice responds with, "I'm glad to know you're enjoying the results of chiropractic care. Did you know that the doctor gets even faster results when she works with children?" For most patients who enter your practice with a symptomatic-short-term-low-back attitude, the idea of treating children will come as a shock, "You mean you see children with bad backs?" asks the patient. Then the C.A. has the opportunity to explain about the birth process being a major cause of spinal trauma that sets the stage for problems later in life. "Do you know of any children who should be checked for this condition?" is the logical conclusion by the C.A.. Regardless of whether the patient can recall any children right then and there, this patient has a new way of perceiving your practice. Should the opportunity present itself, this patient knows that you treat children, and why. So while the payoff may not occur instantaneously, you've planted a seed that may take root at some time in the future.

What if the doctor really enjoys working with difficult cases or patients which the medical community has "given up" on? Let everyone know! Maybe a situation will present itself during a follow-up examination in which the doctor may introduce the referral dialogue like this.

"Mrs. Jones, it's personally very rewarding to see your spine respond the way it has. Have I told you about my special Saturday morning clinic where I work with especially troublesome cases? For the last year, I've been reserving Saturday mornings for patients who have some special condition or problem that hasn't been resolved by other means, such as drug therapy, surgery, problem births, or other cases the medical community has given up on. Sometimes chiropractic can be a big help. Do you know of anyone who has maybe lost all hope for regaining their health?"

Once again, patients may not know of a specific case, but unless you share your dreams with them, they have no basis for describing the conditions you treat or the care you provide other than what they have personally experienced in your office.

If this seems too aggressive for you and your staff, at least make the effort to gently correct patients when they refer to aspects of their care with words from the chiropractic past, such as "kinks," "cracks," and the like. If you don't share the contemporary words and concepts you want used, it will only serve to reinforce patients' misconceptions, halting the advancement of chiropractic.

Take the time to determine the way you want your office and the care you provide described. Ask your staff how they describe what's done in the office! Be sure they understand your philosophy, the kinds of patients you want in your practice, and how to describe what you do. And in time, you will see a new kind of "alignment" in your practice: the alignment of purpose. ■

THE POWER OF
WORD OF MOUTH

It's no secret that positive word-of-mouth advertising is the most powerful marketing tool any business or office can employ. It is the most effective for the very reason it is the most difficult to control. Or is it?

In countless seminars and in-office consultations the common lament I hear is, "I get great results with my patients but they don't tell anyone." How come? Why is it so seemingly difficult to get patients, even those you work miracles with, to tell others about their chiropractic experiences? In other words, how can you proactively generate positive word of mouth about your practice?

What patients think and say about your office is the result of their experiences in your office. And it's not just whether they start feeling better. They compare their impressions of your office, how they feel about your procedures, staff, etc., with the experiences they've had with other types of health care providers. There are hundreds of occasions in your office when patients form an opinion or develop a perception about their experience. These are called "moments of truth." Every interaction they have with your office, from the parking lot to the dismissal process, is being consciously or unconsciously evaluated. Patients are continually comparing their hopes and expectations with the realities they experience in your office.

We all know that when expectations are not met and patients have an unhappy experience in the office it creates negative word of mouth about the practice. "He's a great doctor, but you have to wait a long time." or "She's a great doctor, but they can't seem to get my billing straight."

At the other end of the spectrum, when expectations are exceeded and the service patients receive in your office is extraordinary, positive word of mouth is generated. It's what we all strive for, regardless of whether we sell widgets, serve Italian food, or provide chiropractic care. Positive word of mouth results in a constant flow of referrals and a business that continues to grow and prosper, even in challenging economic times.

Between these two extremes is the vast wasteland experienced by many patients. When a patient or customer enters a business with a certain set of expectations and these expectations or needs are fulfilled and nothing out of the ordinary happens, no word of mouth is generated. It's like the experience we have purchasing gasoline at a self-service station. We want gasoline, we pump it, we pay for it, and we leave. Because we got exactly what we came for and nothing particularly good or bad happened during our experience, neither positive or negative word of mouth about the gas station was created. With this type of neutral gas station experience, we are not compelled to trumpet the virtues of this gas station to friends or family. In fact, we are easily swayed by someone who says outstanding things about a different gas station. Perhaps it is the lack of extraordinary experiences in your office that makes it easy for skeptics to talk your patients out of following through with your recommendations. Providing relief isn't extraordinary. It's expected.

What are some of the expectations your patients have when they enter your office? Most patients expect to fill out some paperwork, be examined, receive some type of treatment, and have their ache, pain, or other health complaint relieved. Sadly, that's about all that happens in all too many offices. You've simply delivered on the expectations patients had about chiropractic when they decided to try your office.

Simply relieving their health complaints will not generate positive word of mouth! What will?

First, recognize that romancing and enhancing the moments of truth your patients experience in your office will take some additional energy and attention to detail. In fact, some of these suggestions may make you feel uncomfortable because of a self-limiting barrier. Here are a few observations I've heard from patients in focus groups about doctors who have inspired ample positive word of mouth about themselves and their practices:

Explain everything in advance. Doctors and staff become accustomed to how the office functions, the office procedures, and even the frightening sounds of the adjusting table drop piece. New patients enter your office quite apprehensive, having heard stories about chiropractic doctors. Patients appreciate having everything explained in advance. Organized patient education procedures can pay big dividends by relaxing patients and making them less apprehensive.

No waiting. While medical doctors can make their patients wait 45 minutes or an hour, since chiropractic care requires many office visits, waiting time is especially important. High volume offices have learned from Disney that even in a long line, if it's constantly moving, there is a sense of progress that can defuse complaints about the wait. Do you keep your patients moving?

Greeted by name. Happily, it's often the easiest human interactions that score so highly in the minds of your patients. Hearing our own name is still the sweetest sound.

First adjustment phone call. Calling the patient at home the evening of their first adjustment has been mentioned in many focus groups. Patients are quite surprised and impressed by this kind of concern. In fact, many doctors take this opportunity to ask five or six questions about the patient's first visit perceptions of the office. This feedback mechanism provides ideas for constant improvement. (Maybe that's why these offices always have plenty of new patients.)

Doctor's home phone number. While emergencies are rare, the act of offering a home phone number (not just the recorder at the office), demonstrates a level of concern unmatched by other health care practitioners. "Here, let me write my home phone number on the back of my card just in case there's an emergency..." Although it may be used by only the occasional patient, the gesture will register high in the patient's mind.

Children's toys. Children of chiropractic patients are often greeted by worn out, hand-me-down toys your kids no longer want and dog-eared copies of *Highlights For Children*. Get rid of the toys with broken or missing pieces and go on a field trip to Toys R Us. Every six months or so, invest in some quality toys. While a Ninja Turtle or two may occasionally walk off, you will be entertaining your youngest chiropractic advocates and sending a powerful message to patients worth considerably more than a couple of $3.95 action figures.

Birthday cards. Yes, a simple birthday card can make a difference. As we get older and the number of candles increase, the recognition we receive once a year often dwindles. A thoughtful birthday reminder (maybe include a free visit?) is easy to do and can make a bigger impact on a person's life than you think.

These are just a handful of the things patients from various offices have told me in focus group situations. Some are quite simple. Others are more ambitious. In every case, the office has systematized the effort so it happens every time with every patient. Sometimes the payoff comes quickly. Yet more than likely, the effort may not be rewarded until months or years later when one of your patients finally has an occasion to mention your name and vouch for you and your profession.

For some, it will always be easier to throw money at a TV station, get lost in a sea of gray newspaper type, or do a mall show. Yet, if you want to employ positive word of mouth from your patients to build your practice, you must exceed their expectations. You must go beyond the ordinary and romance and enhance every moment of truth the patient encounters in your office. Creating situations in which positive word of mouth can be generated takes extra effort.

Maybe that's why it is so rare and so valuable. ■

A CHIROPRACTIC
DISNEYLAND?

My doctor of chiropractic recently remodeled her office. New carpet, contemporary colors, and reupholstered chairs have upgraded the reception room. New paint, wallpaper, and better lighting have given the office a new sense of professionalism. I've noticed I'm even more conscious of what I wear when I go in for my appointments.

Environments dramatically shape the way we think and act. Environments affect our conduct, our expectations, and even our moods. Have you given any thought to the effect your office environment has on your patients? What does it communicate about your long-term objectives? How does it affect your staff? What affect does it have on you?

Sadly, many chiropractic offices that want to create lifetime patients, merely look like a medical doctor's office—a place most patients want to visit only once a year or less. The visit frequency of chiropractic patients alone dictates that a chiropractic office should be more creative, more contemporary, and more exciting than some outdated medical model!

Unfortunately, simply painting the reception room or putting in new carpet doesn't result in dozens of new patients the next day. Environmental improvements are cumulative and the results are experienced over months and years. The effect is long term.

Even after five or six years of successful practice, many offices have the same layout, wall colors, and furnishings of the hand-to-mouth days when they first opened the doors. Furnishings have become out of date, uncomfortable, or soiled. Office literature is dog-eared and void of recent scientific findings. Wall coverings and color schemes that were chosen to be as neutral as possible, now communicate the ambiance of a bus station. The drop ceiling and factory fluorescent lighting give the office a coldly efficient look. The lack of soundproofing and hollow core doors make patients reluctant to discuss confidential health matters. Or at the other end of the spectrum, ominous dark paneling gives the office a heavy, ponderous feeling.

Perhaps you've become accustomed to these familiar surroundings and either look past the flaws or don't notice them. After all, your specialty is chiropractic, not interior design. But realize that your office communicates your self-esteem, your outlook–even your clinical skills. Patients read these signs in the same way they judge a retail establishment by the amount of merchandise displayed, the brand names carried–even the cleanliness of the rest rooms!

The master of environments is the Disney organization. Here are some of their techniques for creating optimum environments. See how they might be adapted in your professional setting.

Many of these ideas were facilitated by Mike Vance who helped pioneer Disney University, an in-house training resource begun in California to train Disney employees. There are three concepts which bear mentioning in the context of the Disney perspective on environments:

Questioning the status quo. When Disneyland was created, Walt wanted an alternative to sleazy, dirty amusement parks. When he conceived of the idea of family entertainment in a park-like setting, critics laughed. Employees would be called cast members. Customers would be called guests. Snack counters wouldn't sell chewing gum so there wouldn't be sticky messes to clean off the sidewalks.

In your office, questioning the status quo might mean singling out paperwork, procedures, policies, or methodologies and reviewing their validity. Do the procedures you used three years ago still contribute to growth, or are they holding you back? Can several forms be consolidated into one? Would you still have a practice if *People* magazine and its pharmaceutical advertising wasn't in the reception room?

Look at every aspect of your office. Does it still make sense? In a rare example of innovation, many state governments are enacting sunset laws, forcing subcommittees to automatically disband on a preset date unless their continued need is demonstrated. We're all creatures of habit, even if our habits are self-destructive, limiting, or result in unseen capacity blockages.

Romancing an idea. Creativity has been defined as inventing the new by rearranging the old in a new way. Often the best ideas are never reached because we give up too soon, accepting the first "right" answer to our problem. Romancing an idea goes beyond the first solution and the individual becomes more playful, entertaining the bizarre and the ridiculous—even opposites. This shows up in Disneyland with Space Mountain, a roller coaster that takes place in the darkness of outer space! Adapting movie set-building techniques makes buildings appear taller than they really are. The thematic uniforms seem more like costumes.

The most important barrier to romancing an office is the fear of being wrong. Of making a mistake. If you were to romance your office starting with the reception area, that critical first impression of your office, what would you do? Would you create a warm, homey atmosphere? Would you offer *Wall Street Journal* for your early morning business people to read? Fresh orange juice? A convenient telephone for making local calls? Moving down the hall, would you romance the names of your adjusting rooms, creating conversation starters by naming them after people who have had an important influence in your life? Would you add more plants or living things?

Funny how so many chiropractic offices that proclaim to be committed to the restoration of life and the unleashing of human potential are themselves dead.

Five-sensing. This is my favorite. The five senses are the only means we have to perceive the world around us or learn about new things.

EPCOT, adjacent to Walt Disney World in Florida, is a great example of five sensing. Here the Disney organization enhanced the guests' experiences by attempting to involve as many senses as possible in the educational and entertainment process. As you enter the front gates you hear dramatic, optimistic music originating from unknown sources. In the Exxon pavilion, you return to the days of the dinosaurs and feel the murky humidity and smell the prehistoric sulfur in the air! At the Kodak exhibit, you see the world's best 3-D film presentation–so real, those unaware of how the illusion is created take flash photos attempting to capture the images! In the China and Canada exhibits, you stand up to see a 360-degree movie that is so powerful there are railings to steady yourself as the whole room appears to move!

By five-sensing your office you can add a dimension to the patient's office experience that can powerfully affect the patient's perception of you and chiropractic. The senses of sight and sound are the easiest. What about touch, taste, and smell? Have you created three-dimensional models showing the phases of Subluxation Degeneration using sand and glue so patients can touch the lipping and spurring as they see it on their X-rays? How does your office smell? Some offices are using the inviting aroma of fresh brewed coffee or hot cider in the reception room. Others are adding small amounts of vanilla or cinnamon to the edges of the headrest paper, changing it from room to room.

The ideas are limited only by your imagination. By becoming aware of all five senses and orienting your office to be more stimulating, you will give your patients a heightened sense of awareness of your environment. This makes being in your office more enjoyable and coincides with the improved function of their nervous system.

By involving more of the senses, we are better able to remember information and recall situations and important events in our lives. Have you ever been in a crowd and caught a whiff of perfume or aftershave that caused you to remember an old friend? The sense of smell is an overlooked and powerful memory device.

What do you want a patient to remember? All too often traditional patient education depends entirely on the sense of hearing during an oral presentation. Researchers suggest that hearing is only 12% effective in communicating an idea or symbol. Add the sense of sight (84% effective) and you have a powerful communication tool: videotape. This is just one of the reasons for using a video-based patient education program in your office. We are visual animals. Video can bring images into your office and into the minds of your patients that they will remember for the rest of their lives. (While we're still waiting for "smell-o-vision," you could use calcium salt tablets so patients can taste the lipping and spurring of Subluxation Degeneration!)

You don't have to turn your office into a theme park, but if you expect to see a patient for months or years, it may need some rethinking. It should have a sense of wonder. It should communicate a sense of excitement and creativity and enhance your therapeutic and clinical objectives. It should reflect the importance of chiropractic and contribute to a patient's understanding. It should recognize that a more normally functioning nervous system has a voracious appetite for stimulation. ■

THE CHIROPRACTIC UNDERGROUND

You have a patient who has been under care for several weeks and their original complaint is clearing up nicely. In fact, your patient is a little surprised at how well this thing called chiropractic works. Especially in light of the cautious skepticism with which they originally entered your office.

But even with excellent results, the patient doesn't tell a soul.

This frustration faces doctors in offices around the country. Based on the "harder they come, the harder they fall" school of thought, it should be the skeptical patients who experience dramatic results who should be the finest referral ambassadors.

Yet, the Chiropractic Underground flourishes. Millions of chiropractic patients whose low, pre-care expectations of chiropractic are often exceeded once under care, don't share their experience with others. Ironically, the Chiropractic Underground often exists in those offices that are seemingly the most desperate in their search for new patients.

I first learned of the Chiropractic Underground from a patient in a focus group I facilitated. It was a group of six "ideal" patients–patients the doctor had singled out as representative of the kind of patients she would like to fill her entire practice with. This patient explained how after he became a patient, he would often offer subtle chiropractic clues in conversations with others. Usually it involved using the word "adjustment." And if this subtle reference were to go unrecognized, he decided not to reveal his own chiropractic identity. Yet, he was surprised by how many people he knew who were under care but had never said anything until he had brought up the subject.

Why are so many patients afraid to openly share their chiropractic experience with others?

Ashamed of their chiropractic decision

Probing to uncover the answer to this question in the focus group setting is difficult. The most frequent reason seems to be that patients are embarrassed by some aspect of their chiropractic experience. Typically it's an image problem. A patient from a Texas office volunteered that he was ashamed and wished he "could park in back of the office." Another wanted to "wear a bag over his head" so no one would see him. These were comments from ideal patients! Even in the face of excellent results, the poor image of the profession gets in the way of referrals. In marketing terms, the referral process is related to something called "post-sales satisfaction," a measure of an individual's satisfaction after the purchase decision.

These closet chiropractic patients are extremely sensitive to the image of the profession and are reluctant to be identified with it. It is as if the baggage of the past and the image promulgated by chiropractic's detractors carry more weight than the obvious results they have received under chiropractic care. Somehow chiropractic isn't "in." Peer pressure rears its ugly head.

If they can't be articulate, or don't understand chiropractic beyond the image on the street, patients risk being associated with the chiropractic of the past. It's almost as if admitting they are under chiropractic care would be sanctioning the "nonscientific" perceptions of the profession; that they had been "sucked in" for a series of expensive X-rays; or had been "swayed" by a charismatic doctor or had used poor judgment by associating themselves with a non-mainstream health care provider. Compound this perception with a low self-image or poor communication skills, and you have many reasons to keep chiropractic a secret.

Other patients say they are embarrassed by the doctor or office itself. These are offices that have not made improvements in their patient environments since the earth tone 70s or when they began practice. The physical appearance of the office and the quality of its furnishings, color scheme, and total image aren't contemporary. It's difficult to proclaim the new scientific findings confirming the importance of chiropractic on one's genetic expression if there's a time warp when you cross the threshold.

Office procedures can interfere with a patient's willingness to vouch for your office, too. If you conduct an aggressive recall program, use fear tactics, force patients to wait a long time, or pump patients for the names of potential referrals, it can discourage patients to tell others. They, in a sense, decide to protect their friends from the same treatment you've dished out to them!

He's a great doctor, but...

More difficult to quantify is the image projected by the doctor. Getting objective input about this aspect is difficult. It's wrapped up in personalities, dress, and other issues. Among the most expensive image decisions male practitioners make is to maintain some kind of facial hair. Expensive because experts suggest that with few exceptions (folk singers, poets, philosophers, etc.), facial hair can measurably reduce believability. It is unknown whether this is a carry-over from the villain's pencil-thin mustache in melodrama or from the rebellious, "out-of-touch" attitude of hippies. For chiropractic doctors, suffering from a public perception that their healing skills are not scientific and their recommendations for repeated treatments are simply financial-driven "opinions," credibility is an aspect of paramount importance. Facial hair, and for that matter, earrings, outdated sideburn length, polyester clothing with "flying nun" collars, or other anachronisms of personal appearance are costly expressions of "individuality" that reduce a doctor's professional credibility.

But preventing the Chiropractic Underground in your office isn't simply a matter of providing superb clinical skills, shaving your beard, and practicing in a stunningly appointed office. It can help, but that's not the issue.

Vouching for you

When patients refer others to your office, they are often more interested in their own reputation than some altruistic, humanitarian gesture of compassion. The question is, how can one of your patients enhance their own position by referring a friend to your office? Or more to the point, how will my relationship with my friend be enhanced or jeopardized by referring them to you? Before your patients can feel confident in referring others to your office, they must consider how well the doctor, staff, and office will reflect on their reputation. How does your office measure up? Have you created a trustworthy environment? A trustworthy staff? Are your doctor/patient relationships based on trust?

How would you characterize your patient relationships? In the report of findings, are you supplying the good news *and* the bad news? Are you quick to refer a patient to another health care specialist if a condition doesn't improve as promptly as it should? Do you encourage patients to actively participate in decisions about their care? Do you put the responsibility for follow-through and compliance on the shoulders of your patients? Moreover, do you provide an organized educational program so patients can make intelligent choices without pressure, emotion, or fear tactics?

One of the objectives of a systematized patient education program is to provide a tool doctors and their staff can use to avoid the necessity of repetitious explanations. Because the question isn't, should you educate patients. Every office educates patients. But how well? And what are patients learning? How long does it take to impart the information and how labor-intensive is it? What are the motives? Is the educational effort being driven by the need to boost statistics? Or the fear that it won't? Is the educational effort being shaded by a short-term perspective? Or is it less than ideal because specific procedures aren't consistent?

Arm your patients

Consistently communicating the Vertebral Subluxation Complex, so patients know their problem is more serious than a bone out of place or a pinched nerve, can help prevent the Chiropractic Underground. You must give patients the words and concepts to help them defend their chiropractic decision and convince others to give chiropractic a try. You must equip your patients with information. Teach them how to conduct a leg length check and how to explain what it means. Teach them how to conduct a cervical range of motion test so the next time someone asks for aspirin at the 3:15 break at the office, your patient can become a chiropractic ambassador.

Your enemy isn't the A.M.A., the hospitals, the orthopedic surgeons, or the office down the street giving chiropractic away for free. Your enemy is the cerebral cortex of every patient who enters your practice. They have some wrong-headed ideas about health and even how their body functions. And unless you can empower the brave patients who *do* venture into your office by conveying the ideas and concepts to promote chiropractic, chiropractic will remain a secret. Forever. ■

MOMENTS OF TRUTH

One of the exciting results of investing in a systematic patient education program is the creation of demanding patients. Educated patients become more critical of knee-jerk medical approaches to health care. Educated patients become more discerning in other areas of their lives as they look to "cause" rather than the treatment of symptoms. Educated patients expect more accountability and ask better questions. When you combine chiropractic care with a regular dose of information dispensed in a non-confrontational style, you change a patient's health attitude while changing a patient's spinal biomechanics.

Chiropractic isn't the only health care profession faced with the challenge of changing patients' attitudes. Imagine the frustration of the cardiologist helping a patient recover from a stroke. More than likely the patient is a heavy smoker. It's estimated that within two years of a stroke, against all the warnings and evidence supplied by personal experience and the recommendations of the doctor, half of all stroke victims who smoked have resumed smoking!

Stroke or not, there are chiropractic doctors (and staff members) still smoking. Imagine patients taking these doctors' recommendations seriously!

Changing ingrained health attitudes is difficult and requires more than a 20-minute report of findings (that actually takes 45 minutes) on the virtues of a natural approach to healing.

Considering patient perceptions, the doctors of chiropractic who are still smoking or are 30 pounds overweight do more than sabotage their own health; they threaten the credibility of the entire profession. The old adage, "physician, heal thyself" comes to mind. It's like the bumper sticker: "Take my advice, I'm not using it."

Finally, equality

Chiropractic faces the same type of challenge women entering the corporate workplace face. To compete, women often must do their jobs twice as well as men to be considered equal to their male counterparts. So too with chiropractic. Doctors of chiropractic must constantly exceed patients' expectations for service, sensitivity, and quality as health care providers just to achieve parity with medical doctors. These critical patient perceptions are formed by a succession of "moments of truth" in your office.

A moment of truth is any interaction with a patient that causes an opinion or attitude about you or your profession to be formed. It starts with the doctor's reputation in the community, shaped by word of mouth, cheaply produced TV commercials, or screaming yellow page ads. It's reinforced by the telephone manners of staff members, scheduling availabilities, fee structures, patient education opportunities, and dozens of other procedures, policies, and office details. It is affirmed on those occasions when a patient has the opportunity to share, defend, or deny his or her chiropractic experience with others.

Those who overlook how patient perceptions are formed reduce chiropractic to a mere clinical procedure. "I just do a better job," crows a chiropractor smugly into the camera and ultimately into my living room in a local TV commercial. I don't believe him. Everything else about his cheaply created commercial suggests the opposite.

Read Jan Carlzon's book, *Moments of Truth*. In 1983, this 38-year-old took over S.A.S. Airlines, the worst-rated airline in the world. He and his managers identified the moments of truth in which passengers formed an opinion about their airline. During the next three years, they set out to improve each moment of truth; everything from curbside baggage check-in to the airplane interiors. The result? Today, S.A.S. Airlines is one of the few profitable airlines around and ranks among the best rated in the world!

172

First impressions

At your next staff meeting, list every significant moment of truth a patient experiences in your office. There are lots of them. Start with the probable tone of the word-of-mouth advertising shared by past patients and even past employees. Try to record the probable first impressions of your location, parking, signage, staff, and office environment. And list the patient's likely feeling during the report of findings, timeliness of the appointments, and the way transitions from one type of care to another are handled. How many of these moments of truth can you identify and then work to improve?

Improving your moments of truths may not instantly improve your bottom line. Like cancer, hypertension, or heart disease, the disease process (poor word-of-mouth) exists undetected long before obvious symptoms appear. Explaining your approach to health and bringing the look of your office into the 1990s won't result in more new patients the moment the paint dries. The effect is long term. Your office and procedures communicate a subtle form of nonverbal language. They give patients important clues about your self-image, social awareness, outlook, and the value you place on the care you deliver. Why should I trust your recommendations or refer my friends when your office looks like a prehistoric hippie-dippy-American-cheese-boring-beige-earth-tone-standard-issue medical office?

Attention new staff members

Patients don't usually volunteer their perceptions of the moments of truth that are weak or inconsistent with your clinical objectives. When they do, the comments are often ignored because they come from your most verbal and assertive patients, the "complainers" or the "whiners." In some offices, staff members are reluctant to mention inconsistencies for fear of losing their jobs. Or their opinions are discarded during the first couple of days on the job when the discrepancies are most apparent to them. New staff hiring policy: every new staff member must offer 10 suggestions for improving the delivery of care and the image of the office by the end of their first week on the job. By the second or third week, the new employee has adjusted to the office, overlooks the grimy light switch, and no longer sees the dead leaves around the ficus tree.

Look for ways to get honest feedback from your patients. Using your list of moments of truth, hold a focus group with some of your more articulate patients to identify the weak areas of the practice. Invite six or seven of your most demanding patients. You're not looking for praise or to hear how wonderful you are. You're looking for the rough edges, the weak links, and the incongruencies in a patient's total office experience. The more "bad news" you can extract, the more direction you have in making changes that will eventually enhance patients' feelings about your office–and ultimately their comfort in telling others.

The mystery shopper

Another idea, used extensively in retail stores and fast food franchises, though rarely seen in chiropractic offices, is to hire a mystery shopper. A mystery shopper is a friend or business associate you trust. Maybe a chiropractic friend or staff member from another community who goes through the motions of becoming a new patient in your office. Their job is to keep notes, recording how they are treated, their impressions, and the way moments of truth are experienced in your office.

Of course this is subjective, but so is every patient's opinion. (Your patients might not be correct, but they are always right!) Start with the first phone call, go through interactions with the staff, and end with the report of findings. Get an objective opinion by keeping their mission a total secret. Have them use an assumed name and call for an appointment at the busiest time on the busiest day. Obviously you'll have to account for the personal preferences of your mystery shopper, but the objective is to encourage someone who cares enough about your success to tell you what most patients won't.

If everything is in great shape, at least you'll have a renewed confidence in your office appearance, procedures, and staff training. If not, you'll have a great "to do" list for making needed improvements.

Exceeding patient expectations

Why question the status quo? Most chiropractic doctors have modeled their offices after the generally accepted medical model. Right or wrong, patients have a certain set of expectations about the procedures, environment, and style of their health care provider. To be taken seriously, chiropractic must outperform a patient's medical experience.

This challenge is even greater for offices committed to providing long-term spinal rehabilitative care. Offices that want to see patients not once or twice like a medical doctor, but 50, 100 times, or for a lifetime, must look closely at every dimension of their practice which might be precluding just such patient commitment.

If you must depend upon advertising, why? If patients are not referring, why? If most patients are not inclined to stay beyond symptomatic relief, why? Sure, it's easier to treat the lack of new patients medically, treating the symptoms with advertising, mall shows, coupons, and direct mail. Yet, when you uncover the cause you'll see the relationship between form and function in a fresh new way. Remember, good will is won by many acts and can be lost by one. Which moments of truth are sabotaging your practice potential? ■

A SYSTEM IS
THE SOLUTION

There are only two types of management problems I've ever encountered in my in-office consultations in the United States and Canada: personality problems and communication problems. These are the underlying causes of virtually every "problem" challenging office growth, patient compliance, or other nonclinical issues.

And while personality transplants aren't likely to be perfected, the real opportunity to make significant practice enhancements lies in the ability to improve office communications. As with all communications, it is the responsibility of the sender to make sure the receiver has properly received, decoded, and understood the message.

The good news is that communication skills are not innate. They can be learned. Like the ability to speak, construct a logical argument, shake hands, or like dozens of other ways we communicate, better communication skills can be learned. Impaired communication is the root of a host of so-called "management" problems:

- [ ] In an attempt to control the staff or the inability to see its long term pay off, the doctor neglects to create a procedure manual. The result is a staff forced to decipher the doctor's intentions soley from his or her behavior. Without mind reading skills they remain in constant fear of making a mistake and losing their job.
- [ ] Collections suffer because the staff doesn't know how far to push or how far they can go and be backed up by the doctor. Can they deny care to patients whose account balance has reached $100, $200, or $500 without payment? Where is the line? The result is

a wishy-washy approach to collections that undermines the staff's ability to collect what is legitimately due.

☐ You're positioning the patient for a neutral lateral cervical X-ray and he asks, "Now, how much radiation will I be getting?" You lie, saying that the exposure is similar to sitting in front of a color TV for several hours, spending a day at the beach, or some other blatantly inaccurate example. And you hope you don't get caught.

☐ Re-examinations don't get done because there isn't a consistently administered scheduling procedure. The result is a patient who feels better and leaves the practice before complete healing is accomplished and for whom there will not be a post X-ray taken to confirm that your technique truly makes structural changes.

☐ When needing to hire a new staff person, the procedure for doing so is re-invented each time. What did we do last time? What questions do we ask the candidates? How do we train the new person? Without a plan, staff turnover and the resulting seat-of-the-pants training send the practice into a nose dive as the procedure is invented again and again.

☐ Patient education becomes spotty or nonexistent because it's too complicated, too difficult, or doesn't instantly seem worth the effort. The result is patients who get symptomatic relief, yet don't understand what chiropractic is and refer to their treatment as "getting their back cracked" and receiving "shock treatments."

These dysfunctional office procedures and many others are the result of dysfunctional communications. It's the "can't-you-read-my-mind?" school of office management. It's "management by brushfire." The doctor's attention is directed to the hottest fire (problem). I call this dancing. The room darkens, the mirrored ball starts turning, and the baying saxophones moan what we hope will be a most convincing tune to sell, keep, prevent, or solve any issue the staff or patients present. Not only is this situational approach to practice stressful, it sabotages patients and staff and reduces your capacity to grow and make the greatest possible difference in your community.

Michael Gerber, in his book *The E-Myth, Why Businesses Don't Work and What to do About it*, observes that one of the major obstacles standing in the way of having a successful small business is the lack of a business "system." He suggests it's the difference between working *in* your business versus working *on* your business. Most doctors of chiropractic work in their business, constantly inventing procedures, standards, exceptions, and otherwise making the simple process of delivering their healing skills much too complicated for the staff. While it is prudent to be flexible and to be able to respond quickly during periods of change, most offices are *too* flexible, *too* accommodating, and *too* vague. There's too much dancing.

When a business is run without dancing, the effect is profound. Do you think McDonald's invents how much meat to put into each hamburger? Do you think they guess how many tables and chairs to put into their restaurants? How many parking spaces? How long customers should wait? How deep the stainless steel counter top should be? What an employee should say and do? Ever see a "failed" McDonald's restaurant? Of course not. It's all in a procedure manual. Nothing, and I mean nothing, is left to chance.

A McDonald's franchise owner in Berkeley, California had a Viet Nam war protest outside his restaurant in the late 1960s. Demonstrators stormed the restaurant, demanding that the flag in front of the store be lowered to half-mast. After consulting his procedures manual and finding no help, yet unwilling to succumb to the mob pressure, the quick thinking manager had his assistant "accidentally" back over the offending flag pole, making the half-mast request a moot point. Almost 30 years later, you will find this solution and many others collected from civil unrest, natural disasters, foreign objects in food, and others all written up in a concise, organized fashion. No wonder McDonald's can successfully open two new restaurants every day on this planet! Does this make a McDonald's hamburger taste good? That's up to you or your five-year-old with a Happy Meal to decide. But it *does* make them the most successful fast food company in the world. What else besides a systems approach to business can account for their success?

In chiropractic, you develop a system so you can spend more time doing what you really enjoy and less time managing, administrating, and handling exceptions. A system is the solution. Michael Gerber invites all small business owners to imagine what it would take to franchise their business. Not that you should franchise your practice, but more than any other "advice," thinking in this way can lead you to some solutions that are systematic and innovative.

Start thinking what it would take to teach someone else to have an office just like yours. Not kind of like yours. Exactly like yours. Without you to coach, rule, troubleshoot, provide exceptions, or be a walking procedures manual. Could you do it by simply photocopying your current "hand-me-down" procedures and policy manual alone? If so, then you're probably doing too much dancing and squandering too much time training new staff members.

Reorienting your practice and systemizing it can start by recognizing those areas or procedures in your practice that remain vague, obscure, or don't get done. At a staff meeting, have everyone list occasions when they feel they must dance. You'll probably discover many of these items lack absolute standards by which to judge their successful completion, are overly complicated, or require too much dependence or waiting on others for important information or guidance. If your staff is in the regular habit of saying, "I'll have to check with the doctor," you can be sure Fred Astaire and Ginger Rogers are warming up in the wings!

If all you really want to do is adjust and spend less time "managing," invest in a procedures manual so your staff is accountable to a written set of standards, and not at the mercy of your mood, your unmentioned fears, or your statistics. Put it in writing. Create a written communication tool that will free you up to work *on* your business, instead of just *in* it. Unleash the full potential of your staff and free them to contribute in more meaningful ways than guessing your intentions. Remove the ambiguities and vague areas of responsibility. Free up yourself and your staff to concentrate on the much more important aspects of patient care and patient education. ■

MANAGING A
PATIENT'S POCKETBOOK

About the time a patient is feeling better and considering discontinuing care, he or she receives a bill for care that was rendered weeks earlier. Rejected by the insurance company, the bill now goes to the patient. And they're angry. Do patients blame their shortsighted insurance carrier? No. They blame you. Because when you accepted insurance assignment you implicitly assumed the responsibility to be a good steward. As a crowning touch to their chiropractic experience they are left with the perception that you have been irresponsible by mismanaging their finances.

Whether it is the result of not paying attention or depending too heavily on reimbursement from third-party payers–pushing each patient's policy to the limit with a super-duper "this-will-get-'em-to-extend-coverage" narrative–the bottom line becomes patient dissatisfaction. When you accept direct payment, you assume the obligation to responsibly monitor the proceedings. Returning to the customer to collect an outstanding balance may work for Pentagon defense contractors, but in chiropractic it leaves the patient with a bad taste in their mouth. Instead of extolling the virtues of chiropractic, they feel double-crossed, thinking they have chosen an incompetent businessperson.

One way to prevent insurance surprises like this is to uncover the formula that each major carrier uses as a basis for honoring claims. Do a little research and find out what each company pays for different types of diagnoses. Do they typically reject the claims at the 15, 20, or 30 visit mark, or do they look at the dollar amount? Find out. See if there's a pattern. Then when patients begin care, draw a red line on their travel card at the visit number where their particular insurance company is likely to balk. In fact, show it to the patient so they understand what will happen and explain why they can't use their insurance carrier's willingness to pay as an indicator of how much care they need. As their treatment reaches the red line, let them know. When it is reached, explain that you'll continue to submit the bills, but they will need to start assuming payment for their care.

Bring your checkbook

Many offices take this a step further by sticking to a policy by which patients, after swiftly fulfilling their deductible, must pay their co-payment on every visit. Patients become accustomed to bringing their checkbooks to your office, just as they would for a haircut, a meal, or getting their car serviced. This also helps combat the perception that care during the Initial Intensive phase of care is "free" because there isn't a direct exchange of money.

This mismanagement is often reflected in collections. Chiropractic is one of the few businesses that has practically institutionalized the idea that there should be a discrepancy, even a large one, between services and collections. Just as poor compliance is the result of inadequate patient education, poor collections are often the result of poor financial education. Combine this with vague or inconsistent policies, and the staff's effectiveness is undermined.

This problem is especially frequent among doctors who have a "soft touch." Whether suffering from low self-esteem or just from being easily manipulated by patients, these doctors modify the financial arrangements privately with each patient. Some even depend on the patient to communicate the arrangements to the staff! And while few offices barter chickens or apple pies for chiropractic care, patient ledgers in these offices uncover a wide variety of fee structures. Not only is this a great way to sabotage your staff, it's a great way to end up in jail! No wonder staff members have difficulty collecting fees!

Offices with high collection ratios run their practice like the business it is. That doesn't mean they expect 100% collections; however, they expect patients to be financially responsible. Forget your checkbook? "No problem, we'll be open for another four hours." Or, "Your outstanding balance has reached $XX, and our policy prevents me from scheduling another appointment for you until your financial obligation has been cleared up." These offices empower their staff by setting exact policies which are communicated to patients and consistently administered. No surprises.

Is there room for hardship cases? Of course. Can you give your services away? By all means. Get involved with the homeless or the destitute and donate everything. A doctor in Yakima, Washington treasures his pro bono work treating migrant workers. Besides the joy of serving in this way, he's starting to pick up some Spanish! The point is to consciously set a financial policy and stick to it. Rise above the notion that if there's money in the checkbook and they haven't come to take away your toys, you're in good shape. Those who merely want to be able to pay the bills seldom find themselves doing anything else. This severely limits their influence in their community.

Could your staff afford care?

A collection problem that often extends beyond the lack of consistent policy, and one that is seldom mentioned, is the staff member who thinks the fees charged by the office are too high. This is an attitude usually found among those who have difficulty collecting money. Staff members, paid just a few notches above minimum wage, imagine how difficult it would be for themselves to pay for the recommended care, and find it easy to side with the financial difficulties expressed by patients.

Perhaps staff members bring this attitude with them when they start their job because the word on the street is that chiropractic care is expensive. And frankly, heavily influenced by the sickness-oriented insurance industry, chiropractic *is* too expensive. For the more than 37 million Americans without health insurance, chiropractic is an expensive proposition. This number will continue to rise as HMOs and PPOs unwittingly suck in more and more businesses keen on cutting health care costs.

Another distortion is caused by the fact that doctors and staff members receive their care for free. It's easy to fit preventive chiropractic care into your lifestyle when it's free. It's easy to philosophically assert that adjustments are worth a million dollars when you don't have to write a check for yours. And it's easy to forget to create an affordable post-insurance, post-symptomatic fee structure in your office when, once a week or so, you're getting your care without any impact to your household budget. Offices that greedily take every dime an insurance company will dole out, without creating a policy that makes non-symptomatic wellness care affordable, have made wellness care elitist and beyond the reach of the average patient. Inadvertently, these offices practice medicine, forcing patients to play the insurance game of inventing a new problem every 90 days or so.

Chiropractic worked hard to be recognized by the insurance industry. Will "dancing with the devil" be its ultimate downfall? Ask the stressed-out doctors with high overheads who got addicted to the easy insurance money of the 1980s. ■

184

THE NERVE SYSTEM AS A MANAGEMENT METAPHOR

Like the nerve system that coordinates the functions of the organs and tissues of the body, your office needs a management system to coordinate various office functions. And like the body's nerve system, a management system can work only when there is no interference. Here are some "neurological and orthopedic tests" you can run on your management system to check for interference.

Consistent policy. Imagine what happens when the stomach has food to digest, but isn't sure it should. Or consider the confusion that would result if the liver and kidneys wanted to trade places for a day or two. What would happen if the heart started pumping in reverse?

The lack of consistent policy is the number one frustration voiced by chiropractic assistants. It undermines the effectiveness of the entire office. Having a written office policy manual is the first check. Yet, having an office policy manual neatly typed in a three-ring binder on the shelf is no assurance of consistent policy! In fact, having a written policy that is not followed is more frustrating than unwritten policies that are at least consistent.

Action step. If you don't have an office policy manual, get one. First, brainstorm the topics that you'd like to see covered and then share your list with the staff. Then start writing. Keep each policy short and to the point. As you write, make sure you test each policy by asking yourself, "How will this policy enhance the function (after all, health is 100% function) of our office?"

Already have an office policy manual? Pull it out, dust it off, and go through each policy and ask yourself, "Is this real?" "Is this being followed?" and "How does this policy enhance the function of our office?" Your mission is to detect inconsistencies between the intent of each policy and the behavior or conduct of the doctor and staff who vow to follow it. If it's not being followed, there's a reason. Often this discrepancy is because the various members of your health care team don't know or understand the benefits of having and executing the policy as written. Maybe things have changed since the original policy was written. New staff personalities may be involved. Reaffirm the value and workability of each policy.

Absolute standards. Running a successful chiropractic office takes more than someone who can adjust and someone who can schedule appointments. And it takes more than "just doing a good job." In fact, what *is* a good job?

What if your heart decided to beat only on Mondays, Wednesdays, and Fridays? What if your stomach decided to digest your meals only partially? What if your lung capacity was cut in half whenever you wanted to talk? If certain functions are not performed to an absolute standard or don't reach a certain threshold, the functions are useless.

What are the absolute standards that guide your job responsibilities? How many rings can the phone ring before it sends a message of disinterest or disorganization to a potential new patient? How long can a patient expect to wait before the wait becomes an issue shaping their impression of the office? How old can a reception room magazine be before it suggests out-of-date clinical skills? How quickly and how accurately should every staff member be able to confirm a patient's account balance? In what way is each patient rewarded for their first, second, fifth, or tenth referral to your office?

Action step. Setting absolute standards is one way to know if we're doing a good job. Without establishing a standard, we simply react to the ebb and flow of daily routine and are always trying to "fix" some aspect of the office. Start timing how long a report of findings *really* takes. Track how long patients *really* wait. Measure the performances of your team so you can establish a standard. Ultimately this will simplify your job and improve patient satisfaction because everyone knows what to expect. What gets measured is what gets done. McDonald's may have "Billions and Billions Served" on their sign, but they haven't stopped counting!

Connectedness. The flaw with many medical research projects is a disregard for a holistic look at the body. Those doing heart research overlook the impact of their findings on other organs or systems of the body. How many times have we heard how the "cure" with its side effects was more harmful than the disease?

To coordinate the functions of your office successfully there must be an "intelligent" nerve supply. This nerve system is the leadership and management direction provided by the doctor, combined with his or her ability to communicate it persuasively. Being an office "manager" is not what many doctors aspired to be. If they could wave a magic wand so all they'd have to do is adjust and do their clinical work, there would be a line at the magic wand store.

Action step. It's human nature to put off those things we dislike the most. Take an inventory of what's not getting done. Narratives? Recalls? Thank-you cards? Re-exams? Collections? Spinal care classes? New letterhead? Consistent patient education? New phone system? Use a staff meeting to develop a list of the things you know you should be doing, but aren't. Then take each item and brainstorm a list of benefits for doing it. How does doing it benefit the patient, the staff, the doctor, the future of the office, or the future of the profession?

If you don't enjoy the management side of chiropractic, consider ways to simplify your practice and systematize it. That's what a procedural manual is for. What do you say on the telephone? How do you trace insurance billing problems? Who reorders X-ray film? When and how? How do you make a new patient feel comfortable on the first visit? What do you do if a patient misses an appointment? Guidelines regarding these and a million other day-to-day activities and procedures should be in writing. Until they are, training new staff members, handling vacations, and coping with rush hours are a constant source of stress and confusion. Procedural manuals explain the "intelligence" of the office so everyone can see the master plan. The growth of your practice and the satisfaction of being free to work with patients and inspire them (the fun stuff) is most effective after your management system is in place.

Outcomes. This is related to setting absolute standards, but also considers the long-range effects of our daily activities. What outcomes are you hoping to achieve by being involved in chiropractic? Check your answer against the seven equities of life: mental, spiritual, financial, family, career, physical, and social. What can you, or should you, expect to achieve in these seven areas through your work in chiropractic?

Chiropractic is more than just getting patients out of pain. That's relatively easy. What are you hoping to accomplish with every patient besides clear up the symptomatic picture?

One doctor I was working with realized he wanted to practice chiropractic for another 35 years. Beside simply improving a patient's spinal biomechanics, he and his staff identified the strong desire to create "lifetime friends" as one of their office objectives. Yes, they wanted to change each patient's attitudes and awareness of health. Yes, they wanted to rehabilitate each patient's spine. Yes, they wanted lots of children under chiropractic care. But the overriding concern was to create lifetime friends.

It changed their management approach. With a 35-year perspective, they modified their recall system. With a 35-year outlook, they made investments in their physical plant and upgraded their office environment. With their newly identified passion to create lifetime friends they found new purpose and clarity in their daily activities.

Action step. Have each staff member identify the outcomes they hope to enjoy in the seven equities by participating in your office. Then, get together at a staff meeting and share them. Celebrate the diversity! Recognize that these fundamental values are what motivate us. Develop ways to help each other achieve these values as you work beside one other. When each individual's values are compatible and reinforce the office objectives, a career emerges. Otherwise your job and your life are nothing more than a series of short-term relationships, empty of meaning and passion.

Awaken the passion in you! Like learning to walk, the first thing you must do is have the desire to move, to be somewhere different. Movement is an integral part of growth. And yet growth, with its accompanying changes, is one of the most frightening things we do. Like learning to walk, we may fail at first. Fortunately, that didn't stop us as two-year-olds, when failure was less important than moving and growing! And we *did* move and grow—as long as there wasn't any interference. ■

THE THREE HATS OF CHIROPRACTIC

At the helm of every small business is an individual struggling for balance—not just the books, but three voices battling for attention. Within chiropractic, these voices are called the Clinician, the Manager, and the Visionary. When these three dimensions are balanced, the business grows and prospers. When one voice dominates, which usually happens in most small businesses, including chiropractic, the business stagnates and flounders against an unseen barrier to practice growth and personal satisfaction.

The Clinician is that part of you with the technical skills to locate and remove the Vertebral Subluxation Complex among your patients. The curriculum at chiropractic colleges focuses on the technical aspect of chiropractic. From the results chiropractic doctors get with their patients, it is fairly safe to say that there is a high level of competency in the technical arena of chiropractic. Of course, there is diversity in technique, but the end result is the same. Why do some doctors possessing superb clinical skills go from one failed practice to another? Because to complement these healing skills and make your exchange with patients win/win you must be a Manager, too.

The Manager sets office policies and implements procedures that are compatible with your clinical perspective and value system. This is the chiropractic businessman, recognizing that fee structures must be set, collection mechanisms established, quantitative statistics kept, and staff management issues faced. Many abdicate their management responsibilities, relying instead on "squeaky-wheel-brush-fire" management. No wonder most doctors have little time or energy to plan the future of their business beyond mere survival.

The Visionary is the entrepreneurial spirit that constantly questions the status quo and reinvents the future. Patient negativity is seen as valuable feedback. Foul-ups are just hidden opportunities. While significantly affecting the lives of their patients, Visionaries don't take themselves too seriously and have a sense of humor about their work that is attractive to staff and patients.

Searching for balance

You'll agree that if each of these personality traits were equally developed and functioning in balance, there would be no stopping your practice.

But how do you achieve a workable truce?

First, look at how most small businesses get into the trap of placing a lopsided emphasis on the technical aspect of their business. While working for someone else, we are given the task of learning and excelling at some narrow range of activity. Let's say you're a travel agent. After a couple of years in the business, you'll have experienced 99% of the kinds of things travel agents experience. You've conquered the computer booking system, arranged tours, handled corporate accounts, and performed a host of other duties. Working at your computer screen, you've mastered the technical aspect of be being a travel agent. After a disagreement with your boss one day, you say to yourself, "Anyone can run a travel agency; look at the jerk I'm working for!"

As you leave with the technical skills of being a travel agent to create your own business, you view the travel agency business as merely a series of technical details. Soon you discover the real truth about running a travel agency!

If you've ever been an unappreciated associate doctor, maybe you experienced a similar scenario. But regardless of whether you started your practice right out of school or worked as an associate first, your technical resources were significantly more developed than the management and entrepreneurial skills needed for a balanced business. And they likely remain that way to this day.

In many chiropractic offices, as much as 70% of the practitioner's energy is devoted to being the Clinician. Reluctantly, managerial responsibilities account for only another 20%, with a meager 10% or less left over to dream in the role of the Visionary. No wonder burnout is rampant among doctors of chiropractic. No wonder the promises of practice management consultants seem so alluring. No wonder so many chiropractic offices look as imaginative as medical doctors' offices.

The challenge is to amplify the Manager and re-introduce the Visionary factor. This needn't lessen your Clinical commitment. Just prevent it from being an easy distraction from facing your underdeveloped managerial skills and the introspection required to identify new dreams for yourself and your practice.

Dangerous inbreeding

If you've worked with practice management consultants, you already know that after the dust settles it's still you who has to assert, confront, collect, educate, organize, direct, and motivate. Yet, many doctors continue to pay exorbitant fees to a parasitic industry that often makes, then feeds off the insecurities (and cash flows) of doctors who no longer see differences in their bottom line or in their sense of satisfaction. Doctors have been convinced to adopt the obscure procedures from corporate giants. Doctors are often exploited even more than they are taught to exploit their patients.

The solution? Admit there isn't a Santa Claus. No one can look after your interests or understand your needs better than you. Look for neutral practice development and business procedures—organizations or consultants not interested in creating a long-term dependency or asking you to change religions. Develop friendships with others who have successful small businesses in your community. Join the American Management Association. Read their books. Attend their seminars. Design your business based on mainstream business thought—not the inbred distortion of someone who was successful (whatever that means!) back in the 1970s and wants to show you how to duplicate it.

When it comes to vision, the last time many doctors utilized their creative skills was when they picked out the carpet color or designed their letterhead. Which probably accounts for why many offices have the same layout, colors, furniture, and chiropractic college graduation photo on the wall as they did when they first opened their doors. But vision is more head space than office space. If you take the time to imagine the office of the future, you can have it today. If you're worried about the future, invent it. Recognize that coasting requires that you go downhill. Without dreaming, planning, and trying new things you assume a passive posture that requires large amounts of energy to react to any changing health care/insurance/cultural/sociological/business shift. If the experts are right, the next five to ten years are going to be very challenging, yet it will be a very exciting time to be in chiropractic. Will you be prepared?

Spend some quiet time each day thinking about the future. Keep a journal to record your ideas and concerns. Read John Naisbitt's book, *Reinventing the Corporation* or listen to it on audio cassette. Write your statement of purpose. List every job function, activity, and aspect of your practice as it exists today and then imagine how will it be done in the year 2000. Question the status quo. What do you want? How do you want it to be?

Just as chiropractic enables patients to enjoy a better balance in their lives, it should afford doctors and their staffs at least the same. This exciting balance is possible after first recognizing what you're trying to balance and then taking action. You can find comfort in Walt Disney's proven axiom: "If you can dream it, you can achieve it." ∎

CONSULTING VERSUS COACHING

The greatest crime in chiropractic is the often complete oversight of chiropractic colleges to give students even the rudimentary management direction necessary to exchange their valuable healing skills on a win/win basis with patients. As private enterprise intervenes to fill this obvious need, distorted values and non-clinical concerns can be interjected into the doctor/patient relationship. The lack of management savvy has spawned an industry which, if the average patient knew existed, would stop chiropractic in its tracks.

If you have a practice consultant, are preparing to renew your relationship with one, or are looking for some outside help, consider these points:

Purpose of having a consultant. Some suggest that the personality and intuition helpful in building patient trust and creating a relationship conducive to healing run counter to good business sense. What many doctors fail to realize is that they are a small business first and a doctor of chiropractic second. Without the ability to successfully run a small business, you do not get the opportunity to truly help patients. Everyone knows a doctor or two who is a great adjuster but who has failed repeatedly to run a practice. We also know of great business minds who perform their clinical routines with bone crushing elegance. Either extreme results in a less than optimum arrangement between the doctor and patient.

Many doctors needlessly sabotage their bottom line and their self-esteem with a lack of sound business skills. One of the fundamental responsibilities of a practice consultant is to help equip the doctor with a systematic way of making business-related decisions. These guidelines should be specific as well as general. Specific, so the doctor can successfully hire and fire staff, provide leadership, negotiate with a landlord, or improve collections. General, so the doctor can appropriately respond to a wide range of situations and not have to run to the consultant with every little problem.

Mutually agreed outcomes. The unfortunate thing about most consulting relationships is the lack of a mutually agreed upon outcome. When a patient enters your office suffering from a set of symptoms, an outcome is mutually decided. Other outcomes may be desired, yet go unspoken. These "hidden agendas" can get in the way, distort behavior, and obscure intentions sufficiently to result in disappointment.

Until these specific, measurable outcomes are on the table, you run the risk of being manipulated, waking up a year later without any real qualitative or quantitative changes, or worse, finding that you've acquired a dependency upon an expensive outsider. It's no secret that the not-so-hidden agenda among most consultants is to get the doctor to re-up at the end of the contract. And while a high percentage of re-ups suggests a satisfied client base, are there continually rising personal or professional goals? There must be accountability. If you just want to be part of a group or feel like you "belong," join a country club!

The consultant's philosophy. What kind of chiropractic "baggage" does the consultant carry into your relationship? What are their interests and motives? What gives them a sense of fulfillment? These are questions usually asked of the doctor and should justifiably be asked of the consultant, too.

Using the seemingly obscure skills of running a business as an entry point, an alarming number of consultants use this opening to indoctrinate a doctor and staff with a pseudo-religious-philosophical dogma that, under any other circumstances, would be laughed off. But packaged with the "Secret to Practice Success" and exploiting an insecurity about business things, these ideas even seem to make sense! Even so, you shouldn't have to renounce your religious beliefs to get the kind of practice you want.

There are worse things than a consultant with an axe to grind! What about the consultant still living in the 60s before the influence of the baby boom generation, HMOs, and an insurance industry increasingly out of reach for more and more people? Or more terrifying, the doctor turned consultant who has based his empire on the "I-had-a-million-dol-lar-practice-and-so-can-you" approach to practice management. Cookie cutter solutions don't work because...

Times have changed. The new patient-building techniques of the past no longer work on the highly-educated, image- and quality-con-scious baby boom generation that dominates our culture. The marketplace has changed, and for the most part chiropractic manage-ment consultants have begun to languish. Countless management firms haven't anticipated the post-insurance environment around the corner. Their clients are being led to the slaughter by being taught to simply do more of what used to work.

Wellness and preventive lifestyles aren't fads. They are sign posts that point in new directions and have important ramifications in the "why" and the "how" of delivering chiropractic care. It's not that solutions from the past no longer work, they're just not appropriate if you're interested in working with the "influencers" of your community and enlarging your practice beyond the frustrating socio-economic group that responds to "free" spinal exams, hot dogs, and Coke.

The only thing a consultant can afford to be dogmatic about is helping facilitate the doctor's individuality. That requires more than just philosophical neutrality, it demands a non-critical attitude. Not just to uncover what is wrong, but to enhance what is already there. That's a significant difference.

Coaching versus commanding. Like chiropractic that attempts to uncover the underlying causes of a health problem, consultants have the responsibility to get to the root of the practice's problem. Treating the symptoms is the easiest way to create a dependency relationship and not make a difference in the doctor's level of satisfaction or degree of fulfillment. Getting to the underlying causes is paramount. In a small, closely-held business, this often means having the courage to admit that the problem is the doctor—not some esoteric procedure or super-duper report of findings. The consultant must have the courage to tell you the truth.

Today, the ability to develop and nurture a coaching relationship is critical to success. No longer is the do-as-I-say school of management effective. Yes, it takes time and trust. Moreover, it often takes resources outside a single consultant to get the job done. In light of the fact that experts indicate 75% of our families are dysfunctional and most of us are co-dependent upon food, sex, alcohol, power, and dozens of other things, an effective coach must be willing and confident enough to refer to other specialists.

Frankly, not every doctor is coachable. Yet, since the highest calling of any doctor is to help prevent what he or she treats, a doctor's consultant has the same responsibility. Look for a consulting firm that wants to put itself out of business. And then start doing business with them! ■

THE ART
OF BEING

"I educate my patients, I do regular patient spinal care classes, I give lots of talks to community groups, I advertise in the yellow pages, I don't make patients wait, and I *still* don't have enough new patients," recently complained a doctor. "What should I do?" he asked with an edge of desperateness in his voice. "Do nothing," I replied, knowing that wasn't what he wanted to hear. "You're already *doing* plenty; the question is, what kind of doctor have you become?" There was a long pause on the telephone. "What do you mean?"

Walt Disney was once asked if he was afraid that a competitor might steal his ideas for his theme park. "By the time someone sees what we're doing, we're already working on the next idea," said Disney. "Someone who copies the ideas of others is always following. If you want to lead, you must trust your own judgment and instincts." Management guru Tom Peters tells the story of the fast-food executive, who, upon touring Disney World mentioned, "I want our restaurants and our environments to be innovative like Disney's." Peters replied, "If you want to do things like Disney, you have to think like Disney." The relationship between being and doing was never more clearly stated.

As a nation, we are taught the value of doing. We are busy people, rushing from place to place in a microwave-drive-up-window-fast-food world. This overachiever attitude has even invaded our high schools, as many students consult their filofaxes to see if there will be time to fit social engagements between after-school intramural volleyball, piano lessons, and a part-time job. There is little time to simply drink in the beauty of a sunset or think about the meaning of life. Are we creating a generation that thinks security and fulfillment can be obtained in the doing of things and the fulfilling of obligations?

Take a close look at chiropractic today and this same phenomena is evident. There seems to be a fixation on the "things" and "procedures" of chiropractic. With the same energy one would reserve for the search for the Holy Grail, you can find doctors looking for the perfect recall letter, the perfect collections script, the perfect report of findings procedure, and the perfect everything. They want to make sure they are "doing" chiropractic correctly. They are mistaken by the notion that if they do it right, they will acquire the joy and fulfillment originally promised in the helping of mankind.

Interestingly, the offices I've consulted with cause me to believe that chiropractic isn't just something that you *do*, it is also something you must *be*.

Procedures versus philosophy

Oh yes, successful offices have procedures. Excellent procedures. Yet, their procedures are the result of a clear purpose and commitment to being an accurate reflection of chiropractic. They are in touch with their personal and professional philosophy. Their vision transcends patient visits and other statistics used by those convinced that procedural improvements are the only way to improve profitability and fulfillment. They don't *believe* in chiropractic, they *know* in chiropractic. "Doing" chiropractic is a way they get to live out their philosophy and "be" an influence in the lives of others. The doing comes from the being.

Virtually every practice management procedure you've heard of works. For someone. Doing a confrontational patient recall program works—for some offices and some patients. Not giving a report of findings works—for some doctors and some patients. Making spinal care classes mandatory for all new patients works—for some doctors and some patients. Treating patients on the first visit works—for some doctors and some patients. Using video to systematize the patient education process works—for some doctors and some patients. Why do some procedures work and others don't? Why do some feel comfortable and others push you to the limit?

Who are you?

When you are clear about who you are (being), the doing part of chiropractic is merely a detail. That doesn't necessarily make it easy. It simply means the answers to common procedural questions are more obvious.

In a closely-held small business like chiropractic, the practice is a direct reflection of the doctor. The doctor's strengths and weaknesses take on larger proportions and are revealed by the office appearance, staffing choices, procedures, patient communications, organization, and the countless other aspects that patients use to evaluate the office. Patients use these "moments of truth" to decide if they "like" the doctor, if they trust the doctor, and if they are going to follow the doctor's recommendations. These characteristics go beyond polished shoes, whether the doctor wears a white clinic jacket, or has an office out of the pages of *Architectural Digest*.

A fight with your spouse affects your practice immediately. However, the impact of a disagreement between a CEO of a large corporation and his or her spouse is diminished because of the company size and momentum. Often it is this highly personal realm of relationships, personalities, and energy level that holds a practitioner back. Not procedures. Not location. Not the economy. It's the doctor.

How do you improve who the doctor is (being) so there can be a resulting change in the nature of the practice? I'm not a psychologist; however, here are some of the attributes I've noticed among doctors of chiropractic who appear to be "whole" and have found a happy and healthy balance between the "being" and the "doing" of chiropractic:

On purpose. These doctors know why they got involved in chiropractic and have a "mission statement" they share with staff and patients. Their primary motive has never been to make money. The money is a pleasant result of being true to a higher calling and commitment to serving others. These doctors have committed their vision to paper in the form of a "Statement of Purpose," revealing the what, how, who, why, and intended result of being in practice.

In touch with reality. Because these successful doctors have a high level of self-esteem, they have created and encouraged advisors to give them the good news and the bad news about their practices. Rather than kill the messenger who brings bad news, these doctors welcome staff members to be forthcoming with patient comments and staff perceptions about the doctor and the practice. You will not find the "Emperor's New Clothes" syndrome in these offices. They hold frequent patient focus groups, use patient questionnaires, and have weekly staff meetings.

Excellent communication skills. They are in touch with their own values and beliefs and they exude a sense of confidence and approachability that patients find attractive. They are active listeners, communicating compassion and interest. They frequently tape record the report of findings, initial consultation, and other patient communications and relisten to these crucial moments with a critical eye for constant improvement.

Challenging mentors. If you want to grow, surround yourself with big thinkers. Most of these successful practitioners are members of "mastermind" groups or search out those who share big dreams. They surround themselves with other "Walt Disneys" of chiropractic. They attend and actively participate in seminars. While they are open to new ideas, their purpose and self-confidence help them avoid opportunity chasing and violent shifts in office policy. By the way, these doctors are voracious readers (or audio cassette listeners), reading books and periodicals outside the discipline of chiropractic.

Long-term vision. Successful doctors look beyond a 90-day vision of the future and look at each new patient as an opportunity to create a lifetime relationship. Office procedures such as recalls and reactivation schemes take on a different perspective among those with whom you wish to have a 10- or 20-year relationship. While they don't succeed with every patient, they attempt to create chiropractic clients out of chiropractic patients. They are willing to delay gratification.

Confront their fears. We all have personality flaws and deep, dark secrets we try to hide or cover up. These weaknesses sap a great deal of energy as we try to keep them hidden. Those who are successfully implementing their ideas of an ideal office have confronted these concerns through 12-step programs, support groups, and counseling. They emerge more compassionate and are quick to avoid the holier-than-thou attitude that can cloud a doctor/patient relationship.

Spirituality. Related to being in touch with your higher calling mentioned earlier, these doctors, while not necessarily "religious," do have a spirituality about them that keeps them centered and in touch with God. Reacquaint yourself with your fundamental beliefs–what would you die for?

Honesty. Simply put, they are sticklers for honesty. Cash payments get recorded and don't find their way into pockets without a complete accounting. They bring out this quality in their staff too. Because they have an "abundance" perspective (instead of a scarcity outlook), they would much rather pay an extra dollar in taxes than experience a single sleepless night.

The bottom line is, these doctors are walking their talk. They take responsibility for the direction of their offices and are slow to blame events in the office on the economy, insurance companies, weather, location, and all the other factors that are convenient excuses. Patients find doctors with this inner-confidence and self-knowledge very attractive. No wonder these doctors have successful practices. ■

THE ALLURE OF
INSTANT GRATIFICATION

Seems that time has become one of the most talked about commodities of the 1990s. Free time, family time, quality time, waiting time, commute time, down time; time has become the new measurement of luxury. The time to relax, time to read a book, time to "be" instead of merely "do".

There are countless books that give practical time management tips on how to get more out of each day and be more effective. Yet, the real challenge in chiropractic is not the procedural enhancements that better time management offers, but the self-confidence and professional image that is projected to patients by one's use of time and vision of the future.

We are a culture weaned on a short-term vision of time. Every evening the air waves are filled with half-hour soap operas that suggest difficult interpersonal problems can be resolved with happy endings in about 22 minutes plus commercials.

Health clubs and diet book authors profit from those who think club membership or buying a book will automatically result in weight loss and good looks. The heaviest and unhealthiest people have bookcases full of these types of books. Expensive running shoes are discarded after four or five uses because the pounds don't come off fast enough.

We neglect to discipline or set firm guidelines for our children, overlooking the long-term consequences of poor character development. We think by avoiding confrontation they will "like us."

Patients fall into a short-term view of their health (pain relief only) and in the process preventive and maintenance care are overlooked. In fact, many doctors overly celebrate the achievement of symptomatic improvement and as a result affirm their patients' short-term vision of health as a destination. Patients end up riding a roller coaster of a series of acute flare-ups. Their monthly visits are mistakenly categorized as wellness care as they continue to invent symptomatic reasons to involve their insurance company.

Wrong tactics

Counterproductive short-term strategies abound throughout chiropractic. Advertising, mall shows, pseudo-research projects, and other schemes look for temporary gains at the expense of professional image and the slow, progressive repositioning necessary to effect real perceptual (and utilization) changes by the public. Whether advocates of these ploys are oblivious to the danger, merely opportunistic, or both, is hard to say. While the motivation to share something as powerful as chiropractic with the world is compelling, the tactics are wrong. Meanwhile, the professional image of chiropractic as a serious health care resource deteriorates.

Some of the chiropractic offices I have visited seem to have about a 90-day vision of the future. Looking around the office, you sense that with a couple of hours and half-dozen U-Haul boxes, the space could be vacated for immediate use by an ear, nose, throat specialist. Upgrade the carpet where the path leading to the sign in sheet has been worn? Heavens no! We only have a three-year lease. Replace the cheap reception room chairs (purchased years ago when price was the major consideration) with something more comfortable? Oh no! That would cost money. Recover the worn adjusting table fabric? Impossible, we're too busy. The aesthetics and impact of these image-sensitive furnishings are often overlooked by those who would rather try a shot at the lottery or invest in the stock market than invest in their own office. The return on investment in your office, while not instantaneous, will always be higher than the best rated tax-free municipal bond.

What is your vision?

What is your vision for the future of your practice? How long do you expect to see your patients? Ten visits? Twenty-three visits? Fifty-three visits? A lifetime? Your expectations affect the way you treat your patients and their perceptions of chiropractic. Things you do (or don't do) to a patient you expect to see only 12 times won't necessarily sustain a long-term relationship. Medical doctors (who are seen only rarely) can get away with 45-minute waits, whereas chiropractic doctors (who expect many visits) must keep the waiting time short. It's the expectations of the relationship that set the standards.

The positive dimensions of fostering a long-term relationship are especially obvious in Carl Sewell's book, *Customers For Life*. Carl Sewell owns the largest Cadillac dealership in the world. Sewell Village Cadillac in Dallas has perfected the art of creating long-term relationships. In fact, the typical first-time Cadillac purchaser at this dealership returns to buy seven more Cadillacs over the next 22 years. Thus, each first-time customer represents almost $225,000 over the course of a lifetime relationship. Obviously, customers who walk onto the showroom floor are treated differently than at the Ford dealership down the street with a sales force interested in simply making this month's sales quota. A $15 misunderstanding in the Sewell Village Cadillac service department becomes less of an issue when the desire is to create a long-term relationship worth thousands of dollars. If the service department manager has a short-term outlook, he might "win the battle" of collecting the disputed $15 and "lose the war" of keeping a lifetime customer. You can't win an argument with a customer, client, patron, or patient.

Similar opportunities are seen in restaurants. The "order taker" with a short-term vision of the future is worried about tonight's $5.00 tip. The career-oriented "wait person" is aware of the positive word of mouth and the hundreds, perhaps thousands of dollars that may be lost in the years ahead due to one experience of poor service.

Living in this short-term world has infected almost every aspect of our culture. Feeding us the images of conspicuous consumption, our most popular television fare is an often unacknowledged accomplice. Are we so insecure that we allow ourselves to judge ourselves and others by what we can buy? The most visible result is a heavily leveraged lifestyle put at risk by the slightest economic downturn. The question is, are you serving the public to service your debt, or are you serving because of your debt to the public?

Spending problems

Spending five percent more than we make each month has become the American way. We are less impressed with the methodical growth of compound interest and more interested in a "win the lottery" strategy. Forget the million(s)-to-one odds. Somehow we think we can escape our lack of discipline and self-created financial predicament by some unexpected windfall. Yet, the squandering of millions by the winners in state sanctioned gambling has almost become a cliche. Most financial difficulties are spending problems, not earning problems.

If you'd like to adopt a longer-term vision of the future and reap the benefits of delayed gratification, here are a few suggestions:

Nurture long-term relationships. Think of every new patient as the start of a 20-year relationship—with or without chiropractic being part of it. Is every staff member you've ever had still returning to your office for care?

Set goals. How many times have you heard it, but haven't yet done it? Still only a fraction of the people I meet have set short- and long-term goals for themselves and their careers.

Patient development. If you're inclined to do mall shows, public lectures, and other public events in your community, frame them in your mind as outreach opportunities, not as new patient gimmicks. See yourself as a sower rather than a reaper.

Visualize outcomes. Not having a clear picture of the result of your efforts is one of the greatest oversights. Imagine the outcomes of faster staff training and reduced confusion of having a procedural manual. Imagine the outcomes and benefits of having a systematized approach to rewarding referrals.

Work with more children. Are you doing your part to prepare the next generation of chiropractic citizens? Attract more children and you can experience the affirmation and almost instant gratification of quick recovery while laying the foundation for a healthier future.

Abandon statistics. At best, statistics are a rear-view mirror look at your past. If you look in your rear-view mirror long enough, you will hit the curb as times change. Recognize what statistics can and cannot tell you, and don't be alarmed by the macro (and usually inaccurate) view that many statistics offer.

Record your expenditures. Spending problems are more easily detected when you record every penny you spend for a couple of months. You'll discover your lack of financial health isn't the result of $200 and $350 purchases, but lots of $12.50 and $25.00 purchases. The little things are what get you.

When you consider the universality of the chiropractic truth and the timeless infallibility of the nervous system (if there isn't any interference), it makes sense to adopt a long-term vision of the future. Chiropractic will survive the insurance crisis. Chiropractic will survive the state legislature tampering with worker's compensation laws. And chiropractic will even survive the short-term-medical-eliminate-the-symptoms approach of the most short-sighted doctors. ■

IT'S
ABOUT TIME

Studies indicate the average doctor of chiropractic will practice 41 years. Greg Stanley of Whitehall Management has observed that each will likely pass through five distinct stages: survival, growth, accumulation, leisure, and retirement. Some of these phases can last up to 25 years or more. Yet why are there so many doctors with just a 90-day vision of the future and nothing more than a short-term plan designed to make a financial killing so they can retire?

Even as a culture we're selling our future short. With stockholder pressure to see uninterrupted earnings, many corporations sabotage a competitive future by refusing to retool or invest in the latest, most efficient technologies. Our steel industry is crumbling, lost to more competitive overseas producers. Our forestry resources are shipped to Japan and return as plywood. All around us we see examples of short-term strategies that mortgage the jobs and futures of entire industries—sometimes whole communities. Merrill Lynch may be bullish on America, but in many corporate boardrooms something very different is happening.

Chiropractic isn't insulated from this myopic trend. But unlike a *Fortune* 500 company that can point a finger at short-sighted stockholders or pressured management, a chiropractic doctor, dentist, or other small businessperson can only look in the mirror.

What could motivate someone to want to make a million and get out of the business unless they had unwittingly created a job for themselves—instead of a career? What would force a doctor to purposefully withhold his or her services by retiring prematurely–unless they had bought into an oppressive vision of what practice should be?

If you were having so much fun you could hardly wait to get to the office, there would be little incentive for an early retirement. Unfortunately, for many this is not the case. Buying into an office modeled after the medical profession, short-term relationships with patients and staff members built on a win/lose arrangement, chiropractic doctors often become oppressed by circumstances.

I get the satisfaction of meeting doctors who are having a great time in their practices, who look forward to Monday morning, and are walking testimonials for chiropractic.

Here are some qualities that distinguish these doctors from the visionless, burned out practitioners who are unaware that alternatives are available:

Enormous amounts of energy. Doctors who are having fun often comment about being "on a roll," easily rising to the occasion of a backed-up reception room or responding to unexpected emergencies as required. If you're suffering from burnout, shake it. Start a physical exercise program and identify some aspects within your practice to become recommitted to. You may need to hire a coach to get you to exercise. Pay someone and buy the discipline you don't have right now. Massive physical exercise is one sure-fire antidote to burnout. Doctor, heal thyself.

Open-minded. More than having a superficial positive mental attitude (lying to themselves), these doctors are quick to entertain and adapt new ideas or generate their own. Yes, they attend seminars. The difference is they frequently go to presentations that have little to do with insurance, technique, or practice management. They are multi-dimensional so they have a wide-range of experience from which to question the status quo. They adapt ideas from other industries and search for ways to do chiropractic better. They are in touch with reality. Because their staff and patients detect this open-mindedness and awareness, there is an excellent environment for meaningful communication fostering respect and commitment.

Sense of purpose. If you've met one of these doctors you can sense they are constantly aware of their own passionate mission. They are trying to achieve something beyond the ordinary task orientation most offices seem trapped in. What's your purpose? If it's to "survive," merely surviving becomes your destiny. If it's just a statistical goal, you'll probably reach it. But what distinguishes you from the competition? Is there anything within chiropractic worth standing up for? Or is it just a job? Big aspirations equal big accomplishments equal big satisfaction. Identify what you would do if time or money were no object. And then do it!

Self knowledge. Do you know your strengths and weaknesses? Doctors who are having fun do. They recognize the importance of personal growth and continue to explore areas of their life they know could offer self knowledge. They are willing to risk what they are today, to become all that they can be. They confront their fears for true breakthroughs. They don't lie to themselves with just positive thinking, they accentuate the positive and work to eliminate the negatives. They're productive because they're constantly growing. No one has ever walked away from a job in which they were still growing. Interestingly, these people frequently cite their insights about themselves as being more important than the arbitrary and temporal acquisitions of cars, houses, or patient volumes.

Creative and nurturing. One of the reasons it's so much fun to meet these doctors is that they don't take themselves too seriously. They have a sense of humor–about themselves and their profession. They nurture others, but take time out for themselves too. So it's no surprise that they are able to attract and inspire a stable, loyal staff. Perhaps this is because they acknowledge outstanding performance and avoid the temptation to punish staff members who make mistakes. They encourage risk taking. They recognize that more can be learned by making a mistake than by a year of seminars. Maybe it's this wisdom that puts a twinkle in their eyes. They are flexible and recognize that frustration is merely a warning sign of an impending breakthrough.

Order and oneness. These doctors seem to have a unity with something larger than themselves. Everything in their lives reflects their primary purpose. They have clean closets. By recognizing that satisfaction comes from within they take responsibility for the quality and direction of their practice. They understand that little can be done to change what happens outside the four walls of their clinics, so they commit large amounts of energy to the experience patients receive in the controlled environment *inside* their office.

Different sense of time. While they are living in the moment they are completely absorbed. Yes, they work long hours, but they turn ordinary events into artistic expressions because they are totally consumed by their work. Their sense of timing allows them to anticipate questions, prevent misunderstandings, and be sensitive to patients and staff. They recognize their leadership responsibilities and set high standards by being the first in the office in the morning and the last to leave at night.

It is this sense of time that most distinguishes those having fun in chiropractic. They understand that times change. These doctors have a deep commitment to chiropractic philosophy that transcends the petty concerns that working with the public always create. They have a faith that makes their 41 years of chiropractic service a blessing to all who know them. Meeting them is an event that continues to make my involvement in chiropractic a pleasure. Have we met yet? ■

NEW PURPOSE FOR
YOUR PRACTICE

Ask anyone back in the early 60s what the purpose of NASA was and they'd tell you one of NASA's goals: put a man on the moon and return him safely to earth by the end of the decade. Why? To beat the Russians who were already years ahead of U.S. space technology. The result? Enhanced national pride. A strong motivator back then.

Like most goals, we achieved them. Now what? What are NASA's goals and objectives now? Their lack of publicly understood goals and purpose has severely limited NASA's impact and momentum. It's more fundamental than merely replacing the Challenger. It's the lack of a clearly communicated purpose.

Dentists, accountants, chiropractic doctors, and other licensed professionals suffer from a similar limitation. Many start out in college with a burning desire to give enormous energy to their professions. After graduation, they begin practicing before designing the kind of practice they really want. Somewhere they are introduced to the real or imagined realities of the marketplace and their previous idealistic vision is choked or put on hold.

The energy necessary to survive and build a practice takes precedence over philosophical considerations, long-term marketing strategies, or positioning the practice for future growth. The primary objective is to get flow—patient flow and cash flow. Frequently this early mind-set sets in motion a long series of decisions that, years later, results in burnout or in a secret yearning to retire and change careers.

Serving two masters

Frequently, doctors attempt to live a double life, keeping their personal values deeply submerged and separated from their day-to-day activities. This separation often blurs the original vision and makes it easier to succumb to procedures that someone says must be in place to survive in today's practice climate. These procedures may be expedient in the short-term, but they shortchange the doctor's career, ability to attract and keep talented staff members, and run a business in alignment with their unique personal values.

We're all familiar with the impossibility of serving two masters. It's difficult to invest your life spirit in a compromise.

The mainstream business community prevents this disparity by drafting a mission statement or statement of purpose. A couple of short sentences that articulate the what, the how, the who, the why, and the intended result of being in business. Many business consultants believe that articulating the mission statement is the single most important job function of the CEO.

But mission statements and statements of purpose are not limited to huge corporate concerns. More and more small businesses are taking the cue and avoiding opportunity chasing and side trips that prompt managers and employees to "take their eye off the ball," and are drafting their own statements of purpose.

Developing and implementing an effective statement of purpose is the foundation for the team effort needed to keep all areas of the practice in alignment. It is a benchmark by which business decisions and opportunities are evaluated. It is a living document that evolves, but clearly states the reason for being in business—and it's not merely to make money! You make money as a natural by-product of pursuing a purpose that is relevant and provides a needed benefit.

Goals versus objectives

It may seem nothing more than a mental exercise to sit down and articulate your values and long-term objectives. But those who recognize the value of "writing it down" benefit by having a powerful new way to communicate their expectations to their staff and creating new focus for serving patients.

This is more than mere goal setting. Goals are important, but then what? I'm sure you're in practice for reasons that go beyond reaching arbitrary statistical goals or service volumes. Goals are like lighthouses you approach and pass as you navigate a seacoast. Objectives are like the North Star, solid, unchanging, dependable. Your statement of purpose should be objective-driven. Your goals are merely sign posts that measure your progress in the pursuit of your objectives.

The statement of purpose becomes a touchstone that makes sure you can look back on your career and experience a sense of happiness and fulfillment. It is a tool for ensuring that your daily activities are in line with what you really believe and want. Is a bigger practice what you really want, or have you bought into someone else's vision of the ideal practice? Would you like to serve more families and children or PI cases? Do you need an associate to accomplish your objectives? Do you need your own building? These and dozens of other questions become easier to answer once you've drafted a statement of purpose. Moreover, they're different for every practitioner.

New staff hiring tool

Your mission statement becomes a vehicle for imparting your "corporate culture" to new staff members. The ultimate essay question when you hire a new staff member is, "What do you think of our statement of purpose?" A flat response is often a tell-tale sign of future problems. Incredible skills without an alignment of life purpose or shared value system almost guarantees a short-term relationship. But if the eyes light up and you can tell you've touched a responsive chord, you have a good chance of hiring a valuable contributor to your practice.

Some doctors are afraid of revealing their objectives for fear that if they really told others what they think or believe in, that they would somehow think less of them. Or that it would be difficult to attract staff members. But just the opposite is usually the case. The opportunity to participate with others sharing similar values is the most powerful form of motivation available. Attracting those who share your vision can create career positions in your office. And it starts with you.

Crystalize your vision

Bringing your "hidden agendas" out into the open can help staff members contribute to long-range office objectives. A statement of purpose empowers staff members to make the right decisions without having to check with the doctor on every little issue. It provides a way to describe to others, even patients, what you're really trying to accomplish.

In focus groups, one of the common deficiencies patients reveal is their inability to describe what their doctor does. No wonder there are few referrals! Their vague descriptions of chiropractic are less than dynamic. No wonder patients with low back problems can only refer other low back cases. If you'd like to break this cycle and broaden the appeal of your services, help patients articulate your vision. Sharing your statement of purpose can be instrumental in enhancing the patient's referral dialogue with others.

The clarification that results by writing it in a sentence or two is remarkable. It's relatively easy to ramble a page or two, getting flowery and profound, but a statement of purpose must be concise and to the point. Take the advice of the Hollywood producer who told script writers, "If you can't write your idea for a movie on the back of a business card, you don't have a movie."

What happened to the sense of purpose with which you began practice? Have you lost track? The first step to recovering your dreams is to write them down. Even the writer of Proverbs recognized this thousands of years ago. "Without vision, the people perish." ∎

REPOSITIONING
PATIENTS
FROM THE CURB

One of the objectives of any office committed to the rehabilitative and preventive aspects of chiropractic is to help change a patient's view of chiropractic. The objective is to enlarge their limited-short-term-relief-only outlook about chiropractic to include a long-term-rehabilitative-wellness perspective. When doctors and staff are successful in educating patients and effectively communicating this view, it shows up statistically with patient visit averages in the 50s, 60s, and beyond. You can see retention figures like these when patients understand a larger context for chiropractic care (wellness), and are more likely to continue with care long after their original symptoms are gone. Changing the perception of a product or service and creating or expanding the market for it by changing its perception is called "repositioning."

This repositioning process, creating a new market for an old service by changing the way it is perceived, works well in the controllable environment of an office. But what about the rest of your community? Those who drive by your office everyday? Indifferent. Skeptical. Confused. Start changing the public's attitudes about chiropractic with your clinic sign.

Chiropractic as a commodity

Even if your business doesn't have a formal name, you likely use the word chiropractic or chiropractor as an identifier on your sign, helping people find a source of chiropractic care. As the general public sees your clinic sign and the word chiropractic, they automatically attribute everything they already know about chiropractic to you. All the old attitudes, misconceptions, and baggage from the past are bestowed upon the office behind the sign. "Look Marge, one of them chiropractors has an office over there."

This same misunderstanding is often faced in the corporate world. Companies conducting business in competitive fields or who seek differentiation of their products or services, use a positioning statement to clarify their market niche in the minds of current and prospective customers.

A positioning statement consists of about four to ten words and accompanies the company name on signage, stationery, business cards, or any other company communication. This short statement is used to amplify, define, or position the company, the product, or service for the intended consumer. Apple Computer modifies their name with "The most personal computer." BMW refers to their automobiles as "The ultimate driving machine." United Airlines urges us to "Fly the friendly skies." The list is endless. These statements play a practical role in defining the corporate mission to the public, helping prospective customers distinguish between competing brands, or describing the corporate scope of work. They position the business in the context of how prospective customers view them.

Perhaps you should have a positioning statement.

There are many types of positioning statements. They can explain, claim, offer a benefit, give a directive, or differentiate your practice from competitors. Chiropractic doctors wishing to appeal to the wellness market often create a positioning statement that explains their preventive services or differentiates their approach from other types of doctors. Those with specialized practices such as pediatrics, use their positioning statements to identify their target market: "Helping children reach their fullest potential." They vary from office to office and reflect the doctor's individual purpose and outlook.

Not a slogan!

While it's short and sometimes "catchy," don't confuse a positioning statement with a slogan. A positioning statement is much more strategic. It must be believable while recognizing the mind-set of the target audience. It must help create a shift in perception. It may introduce some aspect not usually associated with chiropractic. Don't use the valuable space on your sign or business card to merely restate the obvious or reinforce what is already attributed to chiropractic.

Before Apple Computer created their positioning statement, they had to evaluate the marketing environment. They kept bumping into something very big. And blue. Rather than attempt a spitting contest with a huge IBM, Apple chose to capitalize on Big Blue's widely-held perception of being a cold and insensitive company. (Remember the famous "1984" Super Bowl commercial in which they characterized IBM as Big Brother?) Apple's positioning statement, "The most personal computer," capitalized on these consumer perceptions.

What about chiropractic?

Attract more ideal patients

Shouldn't doctors of chiropractic use every known communication tool to enhance the perception of the profession? A positioning statement placed on your clinic sign and literature is an inexpensive, yet visible way to start the process—even before meeting the prospective patient. Moreover, the process of creating a positioning statement can help clarify and give focus to your mission in chiropractic.

Short descriptive statements have been used for years but often reflect a limited vision for chiropractic, restate the obvious, or are simply unbelievable to a skeptical public. Here's how some offices modify their names: "Pain relief clinic." (When the pain is gone discontinue care.) "Total health care." (Unbelievable or unrealistic claim for most people unfamiliar with chiropractic.) "We make it affordable to be healthy." (Chiropractic is cheap.) Even, "Free spinal examination," or "Most insurance accepted."

Many of these "positions" constrict the size of a practice by unnecessarily narrowing the context of chiropractic, its image, or utilization.

What's your position?

Write a positioning statement. Determine what type of services you want to provide and conceptualize your ideal patient. Sometimes this may be different from the kinds of services you're now delivering to your average patient. Some very exciting things happen by going through this clarification process.

A good example is the doctor I worked with who was interested in providing care for white and gold-collar workers: lawyers, computer programmers, entrepreneurs, etc. These baby boomer patients have flexible work schedules, sizable incomes, and are more often predisposed to wellness and preventive care. You'll find these people playing racquet ball at the YMCA at 10:30 a.m. or following some kind of personal workout program. With this patient profile in mind, every aspect of the office was designed with the purpose of being especially attractive to this target market. Office location, interior design, staffing, practice hours, procedures, even reception room reading material were consciously selected.

As expected, this practice continues to grow because these kinds of patients feel especially comfortable and welcome in the office. The crowning touch is the positioning statement, tastefully added to the clinic's sign. A statement seen by the entire community and upon every visit by each patient: Advanced Spinal Fitness.

Certainly this represents a refreshing twist and a significant departure from the just-crack-my-back chiropractic of the past!

Yet, positioning statements are very personal and require thoughtful consideration. The process of developing one can be just as valuable as what you do with it when you've got it. One size does not fit all. Without one, an outsider might think every chiropractic doctor is the same, offering identical services, using similar techniques, and sharing the same personal objectives. Do you believe chiropractic is a commodity?

A positioning statement signals potential patients, reveals specialties of care, and offers clues about the kinds of patients you treat, health attitudes, and other aspects about your practice. It can serve to attract the types of patients you especially enjoy serving. If strategically considered and sensitive to the opportunity of projecting a wellness orientation, it can start changing public perceptions about chiropractic.

Changing public opinion about chiropractic will not happen overnight. Nor are you likely to experience a flood of new patients the day you place your positioning statement on your sign or reprint your stationery. But then ideas and attitudes with real staying power are seldom the recipients of instant bandwagon-me-tooism.

With growing interest from the scientific community and a huge baby boomer market interested in preventive and wellness care, clarifying the role of chiropractic on your clinic sign could pay more dividends today than ever before. It could be a good sign of a healthy future for patients–and the profession. ■

THE SOCIAL
SKILLS OF RECALLS

Ten years ago I met Paul Myers on a weekend skiing trip. At the time he was an accountant working for a large electronics firm. Two years ago I bumped into him leaving the office of a mutual friend. In the small talk I learned that he had changed careers and was now selling computer-generated 35mm slides. He suggested that we get together for lunch.

After 10 years and with little in common, I had no desire to have lunch with him. What would we have to talk about over an hour-long lunch? The only motive I could figure was he wanted to sell me something–probably some of those new computer-generated slides he was pitching to my friend!

To avoid having lunch with him, I refused to set a date on the spot, suggesting he call me the following week to set something up. Maybe he would forget. But much to my dismay, he called. Pretty persistent fellow. Trapped, I hoped to delay it as long as possible and set a time and place for the following week. I dreaded the approaching lunch date.

The morning of our lunch I called to cancel. "Something's come up, I'm not going to be able to make it for lunch," I lied.

"No problem," he said without dropping a beat, "how about Monday?"

I don't want to have lunch with this guy! Can't he see that I don't want to have lunch with him? Is he so insensitive he can't pick up on the signals I'm sending him?

"Monday will be fine," I mumble disinterestedly after a long pause.

All weekend I dreaded the upcoming lunch. Why was he pursuing me? What was his agenda? What was his motivation after 10 years? The more I thought about it, the more suspicious and resentful I became. I was angry he wasn't picking up the clues I was sending.

On Monday I called Paul to cancel a second time. "Well, how 'bout Wednesday," he answered cheerily, somehow oblivious to the pattern that was developing.

After a long pause I blurted, "Paul, I don't think our time would be best served by having lunch together."

Too abrupt? He wasn't reading the clues I was sending him. I remembered this event of two years ago when I recently saw (and avoided) Paul in a grocery store. I couldn't help but see the similarity between my experience with Paul and the well meaning but insensitive tactics often used to urge patients to continue care beyond their own sense of need.

In either case, lunch or encouraging a patient to continue care, the intentions may be honorable and even in the person's best interest, but my perception was that Paul would probably put the squeeze on me to buy his slides. I wasn't interested in his sales presentation.

The wrong method

After years of practice and a full appreciation for the life-threatening aspects of the Vertebral Subluxation Complex, the humanitarian doctor wants to do everything possible to encourage patients to remain under care. The motive isn't wrong–the methods are.

There are a set of generally accepted social skills used in our culture that come into play. At a party, there are ways of excusing ourselves so we can talk to someone else. When we're shopping, we can usually lose the persistent sales clerk with an, "I'm just looking today." Our sensitivity to these verbal and sometimes nonverbal clues allows us to successfully interpret and negotiate a variety of social settings. As valuable as these skills are, they don't show up on the curriculum of any college–except at the School of Hard Knocks.

Missing appointments or an unwillingness to set a specific time for the next appointment are two of these social clues. In "Patientese," they're often saying, "I found what I was looking for when I originally consulted your office and I no longer perceive a need for chiropractic, thank you very much." Or you may be dealing with a dialect that translates into, "The pain is gone and I no longer see a good cost/benefit ratio between the cost of your care and what I'm getting here."

Playing catch-up ball

What can be done to sensitively respond to these messages while encouraging the patient to continue chiropractic care beyond the relief of symptoms? Reacquainting patients with the progressive nature of Subluxation Degeneration or instituting some type of wellness fee structure as their interest is waning might help, but that's "playing catch-up ball" by the time missed appointments start happening.

The opportunity to "reposition" patients beyond pain relief to include chiropractic as part of their continuing health care resources has long since passed. Not that repositioning is a one time event; it isn't. It's an ongoing effort, so by the time the original symptoms have cleared up (and ironically, insurance coverage has ended) the patient has the fullest possible understanding of the rehabilitative and preventive side of chiropractic. Last minute, pressure-filled encounters after the patient has already used the appropriate social skills to say good-bye are counter-productive.

If patients don't perceive the need for continued care, a doctor or staff member's attempt at coercion on the phone makes patients angry. For the uneducated patient, the only motive for continued care is the doctor's interest in getting more insurance money out of the case. And fear tactics have a diminished effect because patients are "feeling fine." Resorting to a "do-as-I-say" approach rarely works with today's better educated baby boomer. And, "The doctor wants you to come in for one more visit," sounds as suspicious as it really is.

First, is it worth it? Do you really want patients hanging around who no longer offer the satisfyingly steady improvement and the glowing "doctor as savior" attitude they had when they emerged from pain? Is it worth clogging the practice with patients who have exhausted their insurance coverage and don't need a full set of X-rays with an 800% mark up? Is it worth replacing the easy-to-delegate-arm-twisting patient management with something more in keeping with the way you'd want to be treated?

Talk chiropractic on every visit

The alternative to these Neanderthal management techniques requires systematic, ongoing patient education. Of course a systematized patient education program is a great start, yet it can never replace an ongoing "low-tech" educational dialogue with the patient. How many patients are missing an opportunity to learn and be influenced by your experience and knowledge because it's easier to talk about the weather and sports scores, punctuated by a few grunts from the patient and an, "Inhale, now exhale"?

If I were in practice and I knew education was the only way to make a fundamental change in someone's attitude, whether it be a health attitude, chiropractic attitude, visit attitude, or payment attitude, here's what I'd do:

Systematize your talk

Since educating a patient is a process, not a destination, I'd systematize the process by outlining a plan in advance so I wouldn't have to invent it in real time. I'd make a list of every major topic I'd want the patient to know: the five components of the Vertebral Subluxation Complex, the phases of Subluxation Degeneration, that sort of thing. That's a quick nine topics. Add to that hypomobility, hypermobility, compensation reactions; you get the idea. Identify 52 chiropractic subjects every patient should know and understand. (This would be good for training staff members to answer questions too.) The idea is to pick a new topic each week (or each day if you're ambitious) and post it on the sign-in sheet or on the door of each adjusting room. "Welcome to the office of Dr. Soandso. Today is Hypermobility Day." This gives the doctor and staff "permission" to introduce the topic in every conversation with every patient. Each patient's health problem would always be related to the day's subject. Patients would know it was coming and expect it. It doesn't lengthen the visit because you're simply filling the usual "dead air" while you are performing your normal clinical routines.

Does this take extra effort? Of course. You've already mastered all the easy ways to build your practice. The "gimmicks" in a growth-oriented office aren't gimmicks—they're hard work requiring the willingness to delay gratification for months or even years. It takes more than a great recall script to build a maintenance practice of cash paying patients! In fact, it takes more than a set of videotapes, a few brochures, and a dynamite report of findings.

Sure, a recall program is easier. Especially if you can delegate it to someone who won't raise a fuss when their conscience tells them they've crossed the line from a professional, "We-reserved-some-time-for-you-and-missed-you" to a socially unaware form of badgering. What type of patients (or customers) succumb to badgering anyway? Ask Paul Meyers. ■

THE EXIT
DIALOGUE

What if every patient you'd ever seen were still under some type of regular wellness care? How many patients would you be seeing every day? Every week? Hundreds? Thousands?

Within chiropractic, there seems to be an almost pathological interest in new patients. And while chiropractic must continue to extend its reach, when it comes to the economics of advertising, direct mail campaigns, and other artificial stimulants used to reach new patients, an improved exit dialogue could help reduce the tremendously stressful process of soliciting new patients.

The exit dialogue is a term used to broadly describe the process, tone, and attitude shown by the office to patients who discontinue care when pain relief is achieved and don't get the "big idea." Most offices train their staff to telephone patients as they begin to consciously or unconsciously miss their appointments. It usually involves an unwilling staff member who attempts to convince the patient of the need for more visits. "The doctor wanted me to call..." or "It's important that you..." etc. Not only is this process stressful for the C.A. (ask them, they hate it!), it's the kind of desperate manipulation that has given the profession a black eye. ("Just like my friend said, once you start going you have to go for the rest of your life!") Ask yourself if squeezing one, maybe two more visits out of a patient will change their overall health picture? Have you ever created a wellness patient by badgering patients on the phone with an aggressive recall program? Probably not. But it forever tarnished their image of chiropractic and your office.

Dear (Patient),

It has been my pleasure to serve you during your treatment in our office. I hope your experience in our office has been a good one and that everyone has communicated their very real concern and interest in your case during the course of your care.

We've noticed you've missed a number of appointments recently and we interpret this to mean you've received as much benefit from chiropractic care as you deem necessary at this time. And while you haven't completed my optimum recommendations for care, we are closing your case file today. While you have an outstanding balance of $000.00, we will leave your account open until the balance of your care has been paid.

We have the unique opportunity to see many patients with a variety of conditions and health objectives, so it is always exciting to see another patient achieve their individual goals.

Please remember we will always be here to serve you should any problems arise in the future. And please call if I can answer any questions or be of further help to you, your family, or your friends. On behalf of my staff, I extend our warmest thanks for allowing us to participate with you in the recovery of your health.

Sincerely,"

Does it seem odd to congratulate a patient for making a decision that short-circuits long-term rehabilitative care? Just remember a chiropractic lifestyle is your objective—not necessarily the patient's. If deep down the patient's real objective was merely symptomatic relief, regardless of what they told you, and that has been achieved, it seems perfectly natural to the patient to discontinue care. Recognizing this, the question then becomes one of whether to extract a few extra visits, permanently ending the relationship, or passing up the short-term financial gain in favor of enhanced professional image, the possibility of receiving referrals from this patient, and ultimately their reactivation when their problem returns.

An effective exit dialogue is more of an attitude than a particular event. Pressuring patients has been a way to "zing" an uncooperative patient or a defense mechanism some doctors justify when they realize they didn't fully educate the patient.

With the available research and scientific findings in existence today, there isn't a higher calling within chiropractic than providing the opportunity for long-term spinal rehabilitative care. While the doctor is always in charge of the therapeutic picture, the patient will always be in charge of compliance. An effective exit dialogue simply echoes your long-term professional perspective and keeps your clinic's front door open and welcome mat out for every patient you see. ■

Service America! Doing Business In The New Economy, by Karl Albrecht and Ron Zemke

Explores the aspects of quality in the service industry for the 1990s. Powerful insights for doctors of chiropractic and other providers of personal service.

Flow: The Psychology of Optimal Experience, by Mihaly Csikszentmihalyi

Some practical ideas to have more fun in your practice by learning how to engage yourself in the moment. Kind of technical, but worth reading.

The Tao of Leadership, by John Heider

This book has been a constant source of wisdom for me as I deal with groups of people. It will help in the mentoring and leadership of your patients.

Why Employees Don't Do What They're Supposed To And What To Do About It, by Ferdinand Fournies

Powerful insights! The title sums up the book nicely. Great for understanding many common staffing challenges.

Positioning: The Battle For Your Mind, by Al Ries and Jack Trout

Pretty much the textbook for rethinking how to present chiropractic as a wellness health care profession.

Dedication and Leadership, by Douglas Hyde

A small book about one's journey towards becoming a Christian from the influence of the Communist Party in WWII. It sheds new light on the process of commitment.

William D. Esteb provides a variety of seminars, consulting services, and communication tools to enhance patient education and practice development through Back Talk Systems, Inc. Call or write for a catalogue of practice aids that reflect the patient-centered philosophy presented in this volume or to receive *The Patient's Point of View* newsletter. Mr. Esteb is available for speaking engagements on the topics presented in this book. Contact Back Talk Systems, Inc. for more information:

William D. Esteb
Back Talk Systems, Inc.
P.O. Box 38218
Colorado Springs, CO 80937
(800) 937-3113